WHO Technical Report Series
919

THE BURDEN OF MUSCULOSKELETAL CONDITIONS AT THE START OF THE NEW MILLENNIUM

Report of a WHO Scientific Group

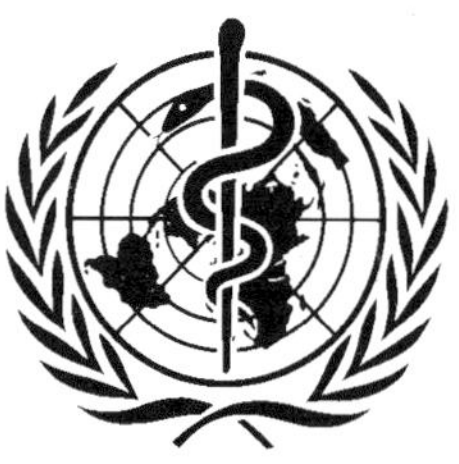

World Health Organization
Geneva 2003

WHO Library Cataloguing-in-Publication Data

WHO Scientific Group on the Burden of Musculoskeletal Conditions at the Start of the New Millennium. (2003 : Geneva, Switzerland).
The burden of musculoskeletal conditions at the start of the new millennium : report of a WHO scientific group.

(WHO technical report series ; 919)

1.Musculoskeletal diseases — epidemiology 2.Musculoskeletal diseases — classification 3.Health status indicators 4.Cost of illness 5.Quality of Life 6.Disability evaluation I.Title II.Series

ISBN 92 4 120919 4 (NLM classification: WE 15)
ISSN 0512-3054

Of the experts who participated in this Consultation, five experts (i.e. Professor P. Brooks, Professor M.C. Hochberg, Professor P. Lips, Professor R. Rizzoli and Professor G. Stucki) declared an interest in the subject matter considered. These interests ranged from consultancies for, the receipt of research support from, share holding in, and speaking at conferences sponsored by companies which manufacture or have another interest in products for musculoskeletal conditions. The Consultation did not, however, discuss any such products, either directly by brand name or indirectly by reference to generic products.

Typeset in Hong Kong
Printed in Singapore

Contents

WHO Scientific Group on the Burden of Musculoskeletal Conditions at the Start of the New Millennium

Geneva, 13–15 January 2000

Members

Dr J. Agel, Department of Orthopaedics, University of Minnesota, Minneapolis, MN, USA

Dr K. Akesson, Department of Orthopaedic Surgery, Malmö University Hospital, Malmö, Sweden (*Joint Vice-Chairman*)

Dr P.C. Amadio, Mayo Clinic, Rochester, MN, USA

Mrs M. Anderson, International Osteoporosis Foundation, Hofstetten, Switzerland

Dr E. Badley, Director, Arthritis Community Research and Evaluation Unit, University Health Network (Princess Margaret Hospital), Toronto, Ontario, Canada

Dr G. Balint, Head of Rheumatology Department, National Institute of Rheumatology and Physiotherapy, Budapest, Hungary

Professor N. Bellamy, Director, Center of National Research on Disability & Rehabilitation Medicine, Department of Medicine, Royal Brisbane Hospital, Brisbane, Queensland, Australia

Dr S. Bigos, Department of Orthopedics, University of Washington, Seattle, WA, USA

Professor N. Bishop, Sheffield Children's Hospital, Sheffield, England

Mr B. Bivans, Coordinator, Global Road Safety Partnership, International Federation of Red Cross and Red Crescent Societies, Geneva, Switzerland

Mr P.A. Bjorke, Arthritis and Rheumatism International, Norwegian Rheumatism Association, Oslo, Norway

Professor P. Brooks, Executive Dean of Health Sciences, University of Queensland, Brisbane, Queensland, Australia

Professor B.D. Browner, Department of Orthopedic Surgery, University of Connecticut Health Center, Farmington, CT, USA

Dr J. Buckwalter, University of Iowa Hospitals, Department of Orthopedics, Iowa City, IA, USA

Dr L. Callahan, Research Member, Thurston Arthritis Research Centre, University of Carolina, Chapel Hill, NC, USA

Professor W.H. Chahade, Director, Rheumatology Department, Hospital do Servidor Publico, São Paulo, Brazil

Dr A. Chopra, Pune, India

Professor M. Cimmino, Department of Internal Medicine, General Medicine and Therapy Clinic, University of Genoa, Genoa, Italy (*Joint Rapporteur*)

Professor C. Cooper, Medical Research Council, Environmental Epidemiology Unit, Southampton General Hospital, Southampton, England

Dr J. Darmawan, Seroja Rheumatic Center, Semarang, Indonesia

Dr K.C. de Mesquita, Panema, Rio de Janeiro, Brazil

Dr M. De Smedt, Head of Health and Safety Statistics, European Commission, Luxembourg

Professor P. Delmas, Research Unit, Institut National de la Santé et de la Recherche Médicale, Lyon, France

Professor J. Dequeker, Catholic University of Louvain, Louvain, Belgium

Professor P. Dieppe, Health Services Research Collaboration, University of Bristol, Bristol, England (*Joint Rapporteur*)

Professor M. Dougados, Department of Rheumatology, Cochin Hospital, Paris, France

Dr K.E. Dreinhofer, Department of Orthopaedics, Ulm University, Ulm, Germany

Dr G.E. Ehrlich, Adjunct Professor of Medicine, University of Pennsylvania School of Medicine, Philadelphia, PA, USA

Dr B.M. Gans, New York, NY, USA

Professor H.K. Genant, Executive Director, Osteoporosis and Arthritis Research Group, University of California, San Francisco, CA, USA

Dr D. Grob, Schulthess Clinic, Zurich, Switzerland

Professor F. Guillemin, School of Public Health, Vandouvre-les-Nancy, France

Dr K. Hamelynk, Department of Orthopaedics, Slotervaart Hospital, Amsterdam, Netherlands

Dr E. Hazan, Attending Surgeon and Chief of Orthopaedic Traumatology Service, National Institute of Orthopaedics, Mexico City, Mexico

Professor J.M. Hazes, Department of Rheumatology, University Hospital of Rotterdam, Rotterdam, Netherlands (*Joint Vice-Chairman*)

Professor M.C. Hochberg, Division of Rheumatology and Clinical Immunology, University of Maryland School of Medicine, Baltimore, MD, USA

Professor O. Johnell, Professor of Orthopaedics, Department of Orthopaedic Surgery, Malmö University Hospital, Malmö, Sweden

Professor J. Kanis, Centre for Metabolic Bone Diseases at Sheffield, Sheffield, England

Dr A.D. Kinasha, Head of Neurosurgery, Muhimbili Orthopaedic Institute, Dar es Salaam, United Republic of Tanzania

Mr A.U. Kuder, Kuder, Smollar & Friedman, Washington, DC, USA

Professor E.M.C. Lau, Department of Community and Family Medicine, The Chinese University of Hong Kong, Hong Kong Special Administrative Region, China

Dr R.C. Lawrence, Epidemiology/Data Systems Program Officer, National Institute of Arthritis and Musculoskeletal and Skin Diseases/National Institutes of Health, Bethesda, MD, USA

Professor L. Lidgren, Department of Orthopaedics, University Hospital, Lund, Sweden

Professor P. Lips, Department of Endocrinology, Academic Hospital, Vrije University, Amsterdam, Netherlands (*Joint Rapporteur*)

Professor S. Lohmander, Department of Orthopaedics, University Hospital, Lund, Sweden

Mr S. Luchter, Department of Transportation Administrator, National Highway Traffic Safety Administration, Washington, DC, USA

Dr E.J. Mackenzie, Center for Injury Research and Policy, Johns Hopkins University School of Hygiene and Public Health, Baltimore, MD, USA (*Joint Rapporteur*)

Dr J.C. Marini, Head, Heritable Disorders Branch, National Institutes of Health, Bethesda, MD, USA

Professor J. Melton, Department of Health Sciences Research, Mayo Clinic, Rochester, MN, USA

Dr A. Mithal, Senior Consultant Endocrinologist, Indraprastha Apollo Hospitals, New Delhi, India

Dr C. Mock, Assistant Professor, Department of Surgery, Harborview Medical Centre, Seattle, WA, USA

Professor D. Mohan, Coordinator, Transportation Research and Injury Prevention Programme, Indian Institute of Technology, New Delhi, India

Dr R. Moser, Association for the Study of Internal Fixation (AO), Clinical Investigation and Documentation, Davos, Switzerland

Professor V.A. Nassonova, Director of Institute of Rheumatology, Russian Academy of Medical Sciences, Moscow, Russian Federation

Professor M. Nordin, Director, Occupational and Industrial Orthopedic Center, Hospital for Joint Diseases Orthopedic Institute, School of Medicine, New York University, New York, NY, USA

Professor H.-J. Oestern, Klinik für Unfall- und Wiederstellungschirurgie, Allgemeines Krankenhaus, Celle, Germany

Ms D. Pattison, Bone and Joint Monitor Project, Duke of Cornwall Rheumatology Department, Royal Cornwall Hospital, Truro, England

Professor R.E. Petty, Department of Pediatrics, British Colombia's Children's Hospital, Vancouver, British Columbia, Canada

Dr G. Poor, National Institute of Rheumatology and Physiotherapy, Budapest, Hungary

Professor J.J.H. Rasker, Department of Rheumatology and Communication Studies, University of Twente, Enschede, Netherlands

Professor H. Raspe, Institute for Social Medicine, Medical University, Lübeck, Germany

Professor J.Y. Reginster, Bone Cartilage Unit, University of Liège, Liège, Belgium

Professor R. Rizzoli, Division of Bone Disease, Department of Internal Medicine, Cantonal Hospital, Geneva, Switzerland

Dr D. Sethi, Health Policy Unit, London School of Hygiene and Tropical Medicine, London, England

Dr T.K. Shanmugasundaram, President, World Orthopaedic Concern, Madras, India

Dr C.M. Shewan, Director, Research and Scientific Affairs for the American Academy of Orthopedic Surgeons, Rosemont, IL, USA

Dr K. Shichikawa, Yukioka Hospital, Osaka, Japan

Professor G. Stucki, Department of Physical Medicine and Rehabilitation, Ludwig Maximilians University, Munich, Germany

Professor D. Symmons, Arthritis Research Council, Epidemiology Research Unit, University of Manchester, Manchester, England

Professor S. van der Linden, Department of Rheumatology, Academic Hospital of Maastricht, Maastricht, Netherlands

Professor T.L. Vischer, Division of Rheumatology, Cantonal University Hospital, Geneva, Switzerland

Professor N.E Walsh, Department of Rehabilitation Medicine, University of Texas Health Science Centre at San Antonio, San Antonio, TX, USA (*Joint Rapporteur*)

Professor S.L Weinstein, University of Iowa Hospitals, Iowa City, IA, USA

Professor A.D. Woolf, Consultant Rheumatologist, Duke of Cornwall Rheumatology Department, Royal Cornwall Hospital, Truro, England (*Chairman*)

Professor E. Yelin, Arthritis Research Group, University of California, San Francisco, CA, USA

Professor H. Yoshizawa, Fujita Health, University School of Medicine, Tokoake City, Japan

Secretariat

Dr N. Khaltaev, Coordinator, Chronic Respiratory Diseases and Arthritis, Management of Noncommunicable Diseases, WHO, Geneva, Switzerland (*Secretary*)

1. Introduction

A WHO Scientific Group on the Burden of Musculoskeletal Conditions at the Start of the New Millennium met in Geneva from 13 to 15 January 2000. The meeting was opened by Dr G. Harlem Brundtland, Director-General of the World Health Organization. The meeting, organized by WHO in collaboration with the Bone and Joint Decade, marked the launch of the Bone and Joint Decade 2000–2010.

1.1 Introduction by the Director-General

Dr Brundtland opened by stating that during the past century, average life expectancy had risen by nearly 20 years, an unprecedented achievement but one whose success had been very unevenly distributed as health and longevity had not been brought to all of the world's population.

The increased life expectancy recorded in recent decades, together with changes in lifestyle and diet, has led to a rise in the incidence of noncommunicable diseases, also seen in the developing countries. Noncommunicable diseases now cause nearly 40% of all deaths in developing countries, affecting people of a younger age than they do in industrialized countries. The epidemiological transition, with its double burden of infectious and noncommunicable diseases, means that many developing countries now struggle with a range and volume of disease for which they are not prepared.

Dr Brundtland discussed non-fatal outcomes, mentioning that although the diseases that kill attract much of the public's attention, musculoskeletal or rheumatic diseases are the major cause of morbidity throughout the world, having a substantial influence on health and quality of life, and inflicting an enormous burden of cost on health systems. She pointed out that rheumatic diseases include more than 150 different conditions and syndromes with the common denominators of pain and inflammation. Examples of the burden include:

- 40% of people over the age of 70 years suffer from osteoarthritis of the knee.
- 80% of patients with osteoarthritis have some degree of limitation of movement, and 25% cannot perform their major daily activities of life.
- Rheumatoid arthritis, within a decade of its onset, leads to work disability, defined as a total cessation of employment in between 51% and 59% of patients.
- Low back pain has reached epidemic proportions, being reported by about 80% of people at some time in their life.

- An estimated 1.7 million hip fractures occurred worldwide in 1990, the figure being expected to exceed 6 million by 2050. Osteoporotic hip fractures account for a large proportion of the morbidity, mortality and cost of the disease.

Dr Brundtland stated further that surveys involving several developing countries have provided valuable information on the magnitude of the problem, showing that the burden of rheumatic diseases is practically equal to that encountered in the industrialized world. She summarized the history of WHO activity in the area, which had its origins at the 1976 World Health Assembly when then Director-General Halfdan Mahler said: "Perhaps the most fundamental difficulty in regard to rheumatic diseases is that the problem is insufficiently appreciated and understood. Critical to this lack of appreciation is an information deficit." Since then, a community-oriented programme for the control of rheumatic diseases has been jointly initiated by WHO and the International League of Associations for Rheumatology.

In 1989, the WHO Scientific Group on Rheumatic Diseases undertook a state-of-the-art review of a very wide spectrum of conditions, from nonspecific aches and pains in joints to full-blown rheumatoid arthritis. The review provided evidence that rheumatic diseases cause more pain and disability than any other group of conditions in developed countries, and the same pattern of morbidity is now being seen in the developing world.

Dr Brundtland referred to a 1994 Study Group that increased understanding of the factors underlying the metabolic changes and considered possible ways of preventing osteoporosis and improving treatment (*1*). Surveys undertaken in developed countries indicated that, by the age of 70 years, more than one in four women had sustained at least one osteoporotic fracture, and the estimated lifetime risk for wrist, hip and vertebral fractures was estimated to be 15%, very close to that of ischaemic heart disease. Further, available data leave little doubt that osteoporosis is reaching epidemic proportions and that it will become increasingly important in most countries as a result of a proportionate increase of the elderly population, as well as a notable change in risk factors.

In implementing the recommendations of this Study Group, WHO has established a task force to draw up a strategy for osteoporosis management and prevention. The International Osteoporosis Education Project aims to improve the diagnosis and care of osteoporotic patients throughout the world, with special emphasis on developing countries.

WHO envisions a way of improving community health through increased collaborative efforts with governmental and nongovernmental organizations. The aim is to increase the capacity of community control programmes to include a wide range of measures, from professional training, patient and family education, and community and patient participation to the enhancement of early detection, and effective treatment and rehabilitation. Further, such programmes should also become an integral part of health services, including existing primary health care systems. An association between chronic musculoskeletal diseases, such as osteoarthritis, low back pain, osteoporosis and gout, and such risk factors as obesity, physical inactivity, stress and smoking, provides opportunities to prevent these diseases through a change in lifestyle. Chronic musculoskeletal diseases can be prevented by including them in a more comprehensive noncommunicable diseases prevention and control programme. The potential in such an approach is great, and WHO is currently developing a global strategy to achieve this.

Dr Brundtland concluded by referring to the goal of the Bone and Joint Decade 2000–2010, which is to improve the health-related quality of life for people with musculoskeletal conditions throughout the world. She hoped that the WHO Scientific Group meeting would build on the foundations of combined efforts and expressed confidence that the outcome would not only be of great value to rheumatologists, physicians and health care workers throughout the world, but would also lead to action to bring relief and hope to the millions who suffer from musculoskeletal conditions.

1.2 Scope and aims

The goal of the Bone and Joint Decade 2000–2010 is to improve the health-related quality of life for people with musculoskeletal conditions throughout the world by raising awareness of the suffering and cost to society associated with these conditions, by empowering patients to participate in decisions concerning their care, by promoting cost-effective prevention and treatment, and by advancing the understanding of musculoskeletal conditions and improving prevention and treatment through research.

Musculoskeletal conditions are extremely common. Osteoarthritis and osteoporosis are particularly prevalent among older people, the number of whom is predicted to increase in all countries, most markedly in developing countries showing an improvement in health outcomes. Disability following road traffic accidents is expected to increase dramatically in developing countries. The question arises as to who will pay for the required medical and social care when, in many parts of the world, the size of the labour force is declining. There are urgent reasons why, in the words of the United Nations Secretary-General Kofi Annan, we must act now.

This meeting was part of a global health needs assessment, the Bone and Joint Decade Monitor Project, which will provide evidence enabling the development of priorities and strategies to improve the health-related quality of life for people with these conditions, relevant to their geographical and socioeconomic settings. The project aims to:

- identify the current global burden of musculoskeletal conditions;
- estimate its future magnitude;
- establish what can be achieved by effective prevention and treatment;
- establish the present provision of care and the ideal provision of care;
- determine costs and priorities;
- establish methods for monitoring the extent to which the goals are being achieved.

The specific aims of this meeting were to identify, review and compile data on all aspects of the global burden of musculoskeletal conditions, and then to establish widely used outcome measures that could be used to monitor changes in these conditions in all populations. The meeting focused on rheumatoid arthritis, osteoarthritis, osteoporosis, spinal disorders and major limb trauma. The problem of children in each of these categories was taken into consideration. Other conditions, such as gout, fibromyalgia, sprains and strains are important but were not specifically considered. Their burden was partly reflected by much of the information collected in general terms about pain or disability associated with musculoskeletal conditions as a whole. Data were identified and opinions were obtained which were relevant to all geographical and economic situations, providing information for the Global Burden of Disease 2000 Study (GBD 2000).

The measurement of the burden of musculoskeletal conditions (Figure 1) requires a model of the course of the different conditions. It also requires data, or a knowledge of the feasibility of collecting data, on incidence, prevalence and outcome. On the basis of these data, best estimates have to be made of the burdens in question. Summary measures of health which can be used to compare and contrast different conditions and are appropriate to musculoskeletal conditions have to be considered, and a consensus on the assessment of the conditions has to be achieved. Data were identified by a wide network of collaborators in different regions of the world as well as by the members of the Scientific Group. A large proportion of the data

Figure 1
Identifying the burden of disease

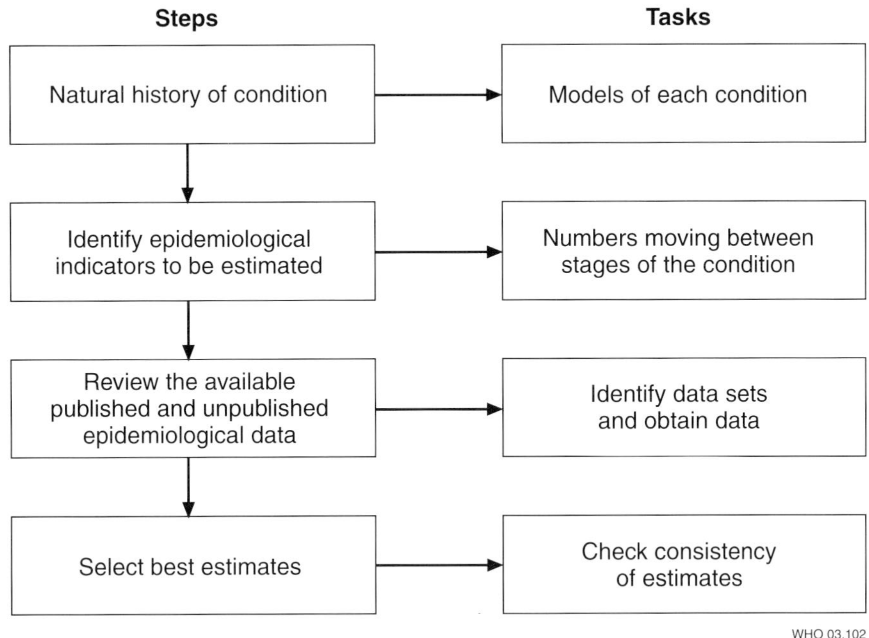

needed was not readily accessible or was unavailable for certain conditions in some geographical areas. The needs for additional data were identified.

The improvement in health-related outcomes requires the ability to monitor and determine whether and how this is being achieved. For this to be possible it is necessary to reach agreement on indicators and methods of application, the choice of which depends on the condition, the socioeconomic setting and the reason for using the data. In this way we hope to set evidence-based standards, establish priorities and develop methods of observing good practice. By measuring achievements and improving care it is possible to gradually improve the outcomes of people with musculoskeletal conditions, thus reducing the burden on both individuals and society.

Certain key activities undertaken during the Scientific Group Meeting are reported in subsequent chapters.

Incidence and prevalence

The available data on the frequency of the index conditions (rheumatoid arthritis, osteoarthritis, osteoporosis, spinal disorders and major limb trauma) and of musculoskeletal conditions in general in different countries and continents were reviewed. With a view to measuring burden, agreement was reached on the preferred disease definitions for the index conditions. Challenges in interpreting the available data were considered. Gaps in data and the reasons for them were identified. Priorities for collecting additional data or for making estimates on the basis of data obtained in comparable populations were discussed.

Impact on the individual, family and society

Data were reviewed and expert opinion was sought in relation to the impact on both the individual and society in terms of the health-related quality of life, resource utilization and social consequences. The courses or different stages of the index conditions were discussed, and definitions were agreed for the purpose of identifying burden. Information from different countries and continents on the health and economic impact of the index conditions was reviewed. The reasons for gaps in data were identified. Differences in outcome between geographical and socioeconomic environments were considered, and possible explanations for the differences were examined. This work is continuing.

Measuring the health impact and economic burden of musculoskeletal conditions

The need for health indicators was considered, and the special requirements in respect of musculoskeletal conditions, particularly the index conditions, were reviewed. Routinely or potentially collected indicators, such as those used for official health statistics, were considered for their relevance to the index musculoskeletal conditions and for their availability in most populations.

The most relevant domains for measuring the different index musculoskeletal conditions were agreed. Methods of describing health status and the consequences of musculoskeletal disorders or injuries were investigated in order to facilitate the development of appropriate summary measures of health. An inventory of assessment instruments for musculoskeletal conditions was developed. Those most suitable for measuring the burden of the index conditions were identified, and their suitability for global application was discussed.

2. Global burden of disease

2.1 The Global Burden of Disease Study

The Global Burden of Disease Study, which began in 1992 (GBD 1990 — based on 1990 data), had three broad goals: to decouple epidemiological assessment and advocacy, to inject non-fatal health outcomes into the public policy debate, and to develop a common metric that would simultaneously measure the burden of disease and be used for cost-effectiveness analysis.

These broad goals were translated into the following specific objectives:

- To make internally consistent estimates of mortality for over 100 causes by age, by sex and for eight different regions of the world.
- To develop internally consistent estimates of incidence, prevalence, case-fatality rates and remission for almost 500 disabling sequelae of over 100 conditions forming the basis on which the burden of non-fatal health outcomes was developed.
- To estimate the burden of disease attributable to 10 major risk factors. This arose because, in epidemiology and public policy, it is not sufficient to estimate outcome measures, but one needs to go back in the causal chain and prepare estimates of the burden of disease attributable to the risk factor. Tobacco, for example, kills people by causing many diseases. Estimating the burden of lung cancer alone would therefore be unsatisfactory. Instead, it is necessary to consider all the damage caused by tobacco.
- To project the burden of disease forward over three decades.

The study itself had various broad components: the goals and objectives as listed above; the need to develop summary measures of population health that simultaneously assess premature mortality and disability; the need to conduct demographic analysis in order to determine the number of people alive and the number of people who die at different ages; and the need to identify causes of death correctly by age group and sex in different regions, as a large part of disease burden is caused by premature mortality. The descriptive epidemiology of non-fatal health outcomes was a major component of the study, enabling the burden arising from non-fatal outcomes to be added to the premature mortality. Health expectancies were calculated, since it is important to know not only how long people live, but also how well they are living. Methods were developed to calculate years of life expected to be lived in the equivalent of full health. In order to measure disease burden and the health gap, a form of summary measure, the disability-adjusted life year (DALY), was used. This is a measure of the gap in the health of a population between its current position and some ideal standard for the whole population. In Figure 2 the health gap is the years lost because of mortality (area C to the right of the survival curve) plus some proportion of the years lived by the population in a state of less than ideal health (area B under the survival curve).

Figure 2
A typology of summary health measures

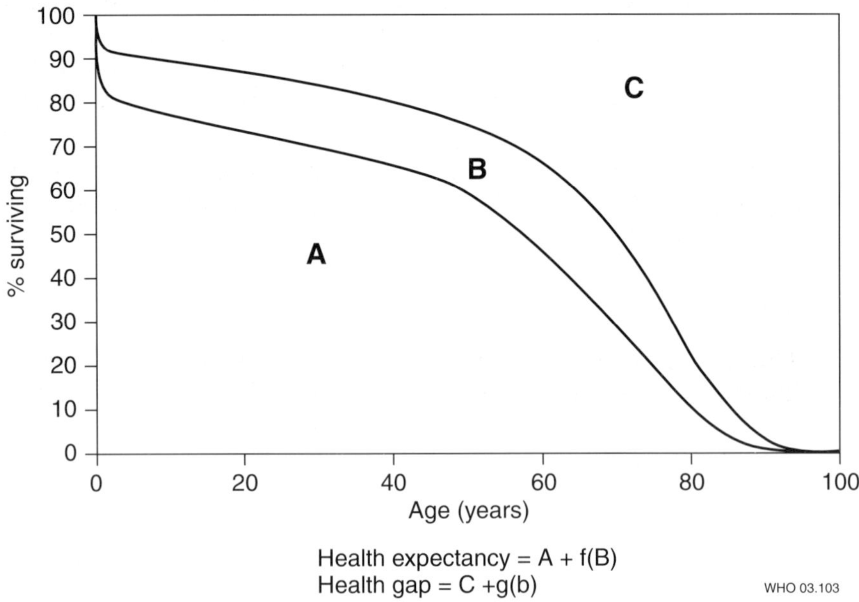

In this theoretical example, area C represents the portion of a population that dies due to premature mortality, area A the portion in perfect health, and area B the portion alive but not in perfect health. Health expectancy is area A plus a function of area B, and the health gap is area C plus a reciprocal function of area B.

The estimates of GBD 1990 were definitively published in 1996. The routine assessment of the global burden of disease is now seen as a key element of the need to provide objective evidence for health policy, and each year an annex to *The world health report* provides an assessment of the current burden. The successor to the 1990 study, GBD 2000, is an expanded project that will benefit from more scientific deliberation on the descriptive epidemiology of diseases.

2.1.1 *Summary measures of population health*

In order to describe the burden of disease in a population adequately, taking into account both fatal and non-fatal outcomes, a summary measure is needed which combines information on mortality and non-fatal outcomes with the aim of representing the health of the population as a single number. This is intuitively appealing but extremely complex from the epidemiological standpoint and potentially controversial, since a summary measure inevitably involves choices associated with social values.

There are some key challenges for summary measures. First, how does one describe health states in a way that enhances cross-population comparability and makes them parsimonious, easy to measure and easy to value? In other words, how are the years of life that populations spend in a state of health worse than perfect health valued? Second, for different conditions, how is the boundary between health and well-being defined? What are the critical domains of health that need to be measured and monitored in order to describe the burden of disease adequately? A parsimonious, critical, small set of domains of health that can be assessed through population surveys is needed. Finally, there is the problem of the difference between self-report and observation in population surveys.

There are currently a number of generic instruments, such as the Short Form Health Status Survey (SF-36), that can be used to measure health status. WHO has used the WHO Quality of Life (WHOQOL) and the WHO Disability Assessment Schedule, but these assess heterogeneous sets of domains, making it extremely difficult to use this type of information for a comparative analysis such as that of the global burden of disease. Work is in progress with a view to achieving some coherence and standardization in these approaches.

2.1.2 *Health states*

The need to value health states is critical when considering the burden of disease. Whom should be asked about this matter? Whose values are relevant? Should the people concerned, the health providers or even the general public be asked? These are key challenges in relation to summary measures and must be resolved.

For GBD 2000 these summary measures of population health continue to be used, but they have been refined. As a measure of health expectancy, disability-adjusted life expectancy takes into account the prevalence of disability weighted by severity. For health gaps, DALYs were used, i.e. the sum of the years of life lost from premature mortality added to the years of life lived with disability (YLD), which takes into account the prevalence, severity and duration of disability.

The estimation of the global burden of disease from largely non-fatal outcomes requires, in consultation with experts, identification of the disabling sequelae for which the disease burden will be quantified worldwide. Experts review the published and unpublished surveys to produce first-round estimates of incidence, prevalence, remission and case-fatality rates by age, sex and region. These estimates must be internally consistent, and this is achieved by means of DISMOD, a computer tool.

GBD 1990 found that the two wealthiest, most demographically developed regions together accounted for about 13% of the global burden of disease, i.e. premature mortality and non-fatal outcomes, where about 90% of global public health expenditure occurs. In 1998, there were 54 million deaths worldwide; the leading causes of death were ischaemic heart disease (13.7%) and stroke (9.5%), both noncommunicable diseases. Human immunodeficiency virus (HIV) was the fourth leading cause of death. A different picture emerges if DALYs are considered, the four leading causes of disease burden then being indicated as lower respiratory infections, diarrhoeal diseases, perinatal conditions and unipolar major depression. The latter condition does not kill a high proportion of people but is highly prevalent and disabling. Road traffic accidents are among the top 10 causes of both mortality and disease burden.

In the established market economies the estimated life expectancy at birth in 1990 was 73.4 years, but life expectancy with full health was estimated to be 67.4 years. Approximately 8% of the average life span of a male born in 1990 in the established market economies could be expected to be lived in less than perfect health. In poorer regions with high mortality the corresponding percentage is substantially higher.

Another important component of GBD 1990 was the risk factor assessment, this being an extremely complex area. For risk factors, the attributable burden (current burden resulting from past exposures) must be distinguishable from the schematically different avoidable burden (future burden caused by current exposures). Risk factor epidemiology is an integral component of the burden of disease study which, using the same metric, allows the disease burden resulting from exposure to be quantitatively compared with that caused by outcomes such as lung cancer and depression. It is no surprise that malnutrition, rather than overnutrition, accounted for about 16% of the entire global burden of disease in 1990. Risk factors such as alcohol and unsafe sex each accounted for about 3.5% of the global burden of disease in the same year. It is worth observing that each represents a higher burden of disease than that caused by conditions such as tuberculosis, measles or malaria.

The final objective of GBD 1990 was to make projections. Models had to be developed for the eight regions of the world. Although data of high quality were often lacking, the models yielded plausible projections. When the 15 leading causes of disease burden in the world in 1990, as estimated in GBD 1990, are compared with the projections for 2020, unipolar major depression moves from being the fourth to the second leading cause in 2020. Current trends in motorization suggest that road traffic accidents will move from ninth to third place. A dramatic change was proposed for HIV, from twenty-eighth leading cause in 1990 to tenth in 2020. However, this projection was made before the explosion of HIV in southern Africa. Estimates now suggest that HIV is already about the fourth leading cause of disease burden. Such projections are extremely important for public policy.

WHO is committed to the periodic revision of the Global Burden of Disease Study so as to provide up-to-date comprehensive assessments of health challenges and needs along with evidence on which to base the construction of health policy. The conference went a very long way towards providing the scientific basis for more reliable estimates of disease burden caused by musculoskeletal conditions. Although these are not among the top 15 conditions, they are important. With better data and more deliberation arising from conferences such as that described here, it may be possible to improve the epidemiological basis for decision-making.

2.2 Estimating the global burden of musculoskeletal conditions

The first Global Burden of Disease estimate (1990) was considered in the 1993 World Bank report *Investing in health* (*2*). This was the first time that a World Bank report had focused on health issues. The time frame for the 1990 estimates was very tight because the exercise was both initiated and published in 1993. WHO has decided to update the estimates as part of GBD 2000, and this effort coincides with the first year of the Bone and Joint Decade. A number of lessons learnt from the 1990 project can be usefully applied to the 2000 exercise.

Because of the time constraints, only two musculoskeletal conditions were considered in the 1990 study: rheumatoid arthritis and osteoarthritis, the latter being subdivided into osteoarthritis of the hip and of the knee. Back pain should have been included, but there were anxieties about the quality of the data available: for many parts of the world there were no estimates of the prevalence of back pain, and the definitions of back pain used in the available studies were very diverse. An unforeseen consequence of submitting no estimates of the prevalence of back pain was the conclusion that back pain produced no morbidity on a global scale. For GBD 2000, it will be important to make estimates for every common musculoskeletal condition and for every region, even if this means extrapolating data from one region to another.

For the 1990 project, estimates of prevalence and morbidity were derived for the eight regions used by the World Bank in its reports. These regions focus on economic rather than ethnic homogeneity. Since a single estimate of disease burden was required for each region, it was often difficult to choose the most representative source. Japan, North America and western Europe were, for example, all included in the Established Market Economies region, yet there is considerable variation between them in musculoskeletal morbidity. Fortunately, the regions for GBD 2000 are less heterogeneous (Table 1). The regions are subdivided according to mortality rate. For each region, condition, age band (0–4, 5–14, 15–29, 30–44, 45–59, 60–69, 70–79, ≥80 years) and gender band, the number of cases, the case-fatality rate and the morbidity rate have to be estimated.

It soon became clear during the 1990 project that the epidemiological and demographic databases for many countries were quite weak. Although some improvement is to be expected, this problem is likely to persist 10 years later, especially as the list of topics for the 2000 project, although still not exhaustive, has been expanded to include rheumatoid arthritis, osteoarthritis, spinal disorders, osteoporosis and major limb traumas. For instance, rheumatoid arthritis has been chosen to be the index condition for inflammatory joint disease. If there is evidence in a particular region that, for example, 60% of all inflammatory joint disease is caused by rheumatoid arthritis, the estimates can be adjusted upwards accordingly. Osteoarthritis has been subdivided into that of the hip, the knee and generalized osteoarthritis. For osteoporosis, data on abnormal bone density, vertebral deformity and fractured neck of the femur will be collected where possible. For the common condition of low back pain, in which it is often impossible to establish a clear etiology, sciatica could be chosen as the index condition. The estimate for low back pain could then be adjusted upwards.

Because the age range for each condition starts at zero, children will automatically be represented for each musculoskeletal condition. Eventually, the large number of studies that focus on overall musculoskeletal morbidity rather than on a specific diagnosis will also be considered. Many of the available studies of musculoskeletal conditions provide only a single overall estimate of prevalence for a given population. These studies are of limited use, particularly when it comes to extrapolating to other populations or making future projections, for which age-specific and gender-specific estimates of prevalence and morbidity are needed. Even studies that provide such estimates often have "empty" cells. If, when a population survey is

Table 1
Regional categories for GBD 2000

WHO Region	Mortality stratum[a]	WHO Member States
African Region	D	Algeria, Angola, Benin, Burkina Faso, Cameroon, Cape Verde, Chad, Comoros, Equatorial Guinea, Gabon, Gambia, Ghana, Guinea, Guinea-Bissau, Liberia, Madagascar, Mali, Mauritania, Mauritius, Niger, Nigeria, Sao Tome and Principe, Senegal, Seychelles, Sierra Leone, Togo
	E	Botswana, Burundi, Central African Republic, Congo, Côte d'Ivoire, Eritrea, Ethiopia, Kenya, Lesotho, Malawi, Mozambique, Namibia, Rwanda, South Africa, Swaziland, Uganda, United Republic of Tanzania, Zambia, Zimbabwe
Region of the Americas	A	Canada, Cuba, United States of America
	B	Antigua and Barbuda, Argentina, Bahamas, Barbados, Belize, Brazil, Chile, Colombia, Costa Rica, Dominica, Dominican Republic, El Salvador, Grenada, Guyana, Honduras, Jamaica, Mexico, Panama, Paraguay, Saint Kitts and Nevis, Saint Lucia, Saint Vincent and the Grenadines, Suriname, Trinidad and Tobago, Uruguay, Venezuela
	D	Bolivia, Ecuador, Guatemala, Haiti, Nicaragua, Peru
South-East Asia Region	B	Indonesia, Sri Lanka, Thailand
	D	Bangladesh, Bhutan, Democratic People's Republic of Korea, India, Maldives, Myanmar, Nepal
European Region	A	Andorra, Austria, Belgium, Croatia, Czech Republic, Denmark, Finland, France, Germany, Greece, Iceland, Ireland, Israel, Italy, Luxembourg, Malta, Monaco, Netherlands, Norway, Portugal, San Marino, Slovenia, Spain, Sweden, Switzerland, United Kingdom
	B	Albania, Armenia, Azerbaijan, Bosnia and Herzegovina, Bulgaria, Georgia, Kyrgyzstan, Poland, Romania, Serbia and Montenegro, Slovakia, Tajikistan, The former Yugoslav Republic of Macedonia, Turkey, Turkmenistan, Uzbekistan
	C	Belarus, Estonia, Hungary, Kazakhstan, Latvia, Lithuania, Republic of Moldova, Russian Federation, Ukraine
Eastern Mediterranean Region	B	Bahrain, Cyprus, Iran, Jordan, Kuwait, Lebanon, Libyan Arab Jamahiriya, Oman, Qatar, Saudi Arabia, Syrian Arab Republic, Tunisia, United Arab Emirates
	D	Afghanistan, Djibouti, Egypt, Iraq, Morocco, Pakistan, Somalia, Sudan, Yemen
Western Pacific Region	A	Australia, Brunei Darussalam, Japan, New Zealand, Singapore

Table 1 (*Continued*)

WHO Region	Mortality stratum[a]	WHO Member States
	B	Cambodia, China, Cook Islands, Federated States of Micronesia, Fiji, Kiribati, Lao People's Democratic Republic, Malaysia, Marshall Islands, Mongolia, Nauru, Niue, Palau, Papua New Guinea, Philippines, Republic of Korea, Samoa, Solomon Islands, Tonga, Tuvalu, Vanuatu, Viet Nam

[a] A = very low child mortality, very low adult mortality; B = low child mortality, low adult mortality; C = low child mortality, high adult mortality; D = high child mortality, high adult mortality; E = high child mortality, very high adult mortality.

conducted, no cases of a condition are found in a particular age group, the logical conclusion is that the prevalence in that age group is zero. In the Global Burden of Disease Studies, one needs to "smooth" the estimates in order to provide internally consistent results.

In putting together a global picture of a particular condition, it would be desirable to use studies employing the same case definition. Most studies of rheumatoid arthritis use a standardized case definition, but with back pain almost every study has a definition of its own. This may account for the apparently major differences globally in the prevalence of back pain; studies that ask about back pain lasting for one week or more are, for example, bound to produce a higher estimate of prevalence than those asking about back pain lasting for one or more months. The explanation here is that back pain is largely self-healing, so the traditional model of systemic diseases does not fit the common ailment of unspecific pain in the musculoskeletal system. The course of disease is different and must be understood.

As part of GBD 1990, the DISMOD computer program was developed to ensure consistency between estimates of incidence, prevalence, remission and case-fatality rates for a disease in a population. When not all epidemiological parameters are available, DISMOD can also be used to model prevalence from estimates of incidence, remission and case fatality or to model incidence from estimates of prevalence, remission and case fatality. Most epidemiological studies of musculoskeletal conditions focus on prevalence rather than incidence; if estimates of remission rates (either spontaneous or attributable to surgical or medical interventions) and case-fatality rates can be made, DISMOD can be used to estimate age-specific and sex-specific incidence rates for these conditions.

The 2000 project aims to produce estimates of the global burden of disease that are consistent among diseases. In other words the number of deaths attributed to each condition should add up to the total number of deaths. Each death can currently be attributed only to a single cause, which may lead to an underestimate of the burden of musculoskeletal conditions. There is evidence, for example, that rheumatoid arthritis and systemic lupus erythematosus are associated with an increased mortality from infection and from ischaemic heart disease. In the Global Burden of Disease Studies, these deaths are attributed solely to infectious diseases or coronary artery disease respectively, yet the individuals in question might have lived for a further 10 or 20 years had they not had the musculoskeletal condition as a comorbidity.

The issue of "double counting" within the musculoskeletal estimates must also be addressed. Most published studies focus on single symptoms, estimating, for example, the prevalence of knee pain or back pain, yet many individuals have both. If the estimates for each musculoskeletal condition are simply added up, there will be an overestimate of the total number of individuals affected.

Estimating the number of cases of a particular condition is the easier part of the Global Burden of Disease Studies; the more difficult part involves estimating the burden of disability experienced by the individuals concerned. Some people have mild disease, while others have severe disease. At any given time, disease will have developed very recently in some people, whereas in others it will have been present for many years. So how does one estimate and quantify the lifetime of disability that a person developing rheumatoid arthritis today will experience? How does one estimate the disability of an individual with persistent low back pain and comorbidities such as diabetes and depression, given that comorbidity and a musculoskeletal condition can greatly affect disability? Most such questions have to be answered by experts coming to agreed judgements, since there are very few published longitudinal data on any of the conditions under consideration, and the few studies available all come from developed countries. There is little information on the course and prognosis of musculoskeletal conditions in developing countries. It is helpful, at the beginning of the Bone and Joint Decade, to know where the major deficiencies of knowledge exist. There will then be a decade of opportunity in which to fill the gaps in knowledge and work towards diminishing the global burden of musculoskeletal conditions.

In summary, the goal of the Scientific Group was to identify, obtain and amalgamate studies on the prevalence and incidence of the five index musculoskeletal conditions from all parts of the globe. Information on the course of these index conditions with regard to remission rate, accumulated disability and mortality rate would also be sought. Finally, attempts would be made to identify information on the severity of these conditions in different parts of the world.

2.3 Methodology of estimating the burden of disease

WHO's two main objectives for GBD 2000 are to establish internally consistent estimates of:

— mortality by age, sex and region for over 150 diseases and injuries;
— incidence, prevalence, case-fatality rates and duration by age, sex and region for approximately 500 disabling sequelae.

As a measure of outcome in the analysis of health systems performance for WHO Member States, this study will provide a clearer picture of patterns of health in different regions as inputs to the setting of priorities for health systems, international public health endeavours and health research (*3*, *4*).

The estimation of YLD is the most difficult component of GBD 2000. Whereas information on causes of death largely relies on one data source, the estimation of YLD depends on a wide range of data sources specific to each disease (*5*). This requires a judgement to be made as to the most plausible source of information and the parameters best describing the disability caused by each disease. The basis of this is a good understanding of the epidemiology of the disease. Creativity and plausibility are essential in assessing and using the evidence.

There are three phases in the epidemiological description of non-fatal outcomes (*6*). The first relates to the systematic review of current knowledge of the selected disease and its sequelae. From this, a diagram of the natural history of the disease or the course of the condition and sequelae is constructed. Epidemiological indicators requiring estimation are identified, for which purpose published and unpublished epidemiological data have to be identified, and material relating to health surveys, hospital discharges and epidemiological studies has to be collated.

Various models can be created from this information. They may include outcomes and consequences as well as risk factors. Such models should identify the different stages of any condition, giving definitions and levels of severity and disability. The probabilities of being in or of moving between stages should be estimated.

The data required to estimate YLD concern disability incidence, disability duration, age at onset (if age weights are applied) and distribution by severity class, all of which must be disaggregated by age and sex. These in turn require estimates of incidence, remission, case-fatality rates or relative risk, by both age and sex. Information on incidence and duration is not available for most diseases. As a rule there is information on prevalence or disabling sequelae. The estimation of incidence and average duration from prevalence figures requires additional information on remission and case-fatality rates or on the relative risk of mortality.

Various diseases that are a significant cause of disability occur at very different levels of severity. Such diseases include depression, anxiety disorders, dementia, chronic obstructive pulmonary disease and arthritis, all of which can present with symptoms that range from being mild to very severe. GBD 1990 determined a distribution of each condition in the treated and untreated form across seven disability classes for each of five age groups. A single disability weight was obtained for treated and untreated forms of each disease by multiplying the percentage in each class by the corresponding disability weight defining the class. After the percentage of persons receiving treatment in each region had been estimated, the overall disability for a particular condition and region was deduced. A similar approach is being used in GBD 2000.

There are many different data sources, both published and unpublished, that should be scrutinized in order to develop burden of disease estimates for non-fatal conditions. Health facility data, which traditionally tend to be reported in connection with epidemiological surveillance activities, are not a very useful source of information for conditions such as musculoskeletal disorders.

Health interview surveys of the general population can provide self-reported information on conditions and disabilities in key domains such as self-care, occupation or recreation, but such information is usually highly problematic. It is often difficult to attribute impairment to the underlying causes. Moreover, there are often considerable differences between the disease concept held by the general public and the medically defined disease category for which information is required. Surveys of osteoarthritis tend to report prevalence figures that are much higher than those obtained in studies employing clinical and radiological criteria to distinguish osteoarthritis from other conditions that cause joint pain.

If information from surveys of good quality is lacking, the next most useful source tends to be epidemiological studies. In particular, longitudinal studies of the natural history of a disease can provide a wealth of information on its incidence, average duration, severity, and remission and case-fatality rates. However, such studies are rare because they are very costly. As they are often conducted in a particular region or town, the parameters for extrapolating the results to the whole population must be carefully considered. For most diseases, so little is known about parameters such as remission, relative risk of dying and average duration that YLD calculations tend to rely on the few studies that have provided estimates of them.

Care has to be taken not only in considering which sources to employ but also in ensuring the comparability of the information used and the quality of the studies so that burden of disease estimates are transparent and accountable.

The second phase of the epidemiological description of non-fatal outcomes involves checking the internal consistency of the information that is being gathered and adjusting the data for non-representativeness. This must be an interactive process with constant expert consultation. It is also necessary to revise the estimates regularly.

Analysing whether disparate sources of information on prevalence, incidence and mortality are consistent with each other requires the aid of a computer. The DISMOD software makes it possible to check whether a set of assumptions on incidence, prevalence, remission, case-fatality rates and observed mortality figures are consistent with one another. DISMOD simulates the epidemiology of a disease in a population by solving a set of differential equations that characterize the transition between susceptible individuals, cases and deaths. Usually, the available data are not consistent with each other, and a judgement has to be made as to which data source is most likely to represent the real situation in a given community.

The only data available on a particular disability may be clearly biased. For example, skin test data for tuberculosis may only be available for a region known to be much more economically advanced than the rest of a country. In such a situation the estimates of incidence and duration must be adjusted to take account of the expected epidemiological variation in the community. It may also be necessary to take into account that access to treatment is greater in the study area than elsewhere and to assume, therefore, that the case-fatality rate for the whole population is higher than that for the study area.

When such adjustments have to be made, the logic underlying them should be presented and justified to national and, if necessary, international experts in the disease area, and should be the subject of consultation with them. Consultations with experts are essential on estimates of incidence, prevalence, age of onset and duration of disability. The consultation process can uncover unused data sources, identify computational and analytical mistakes, and broaden participation in the study. Perhaps the greatest challenge is that the traditional epidemiological models do not apply to the most common musculoskeletal conditions, e.g. nonspecific pain in the back, neck and/or knee. Psychological and psychosocial factors are far more predictive of disability than the medical conditions themselves. An adjustment must therefore be made from traditional models towards a more inclusive biopsychosocial model for musculoskeletal disorders (7).

The role of the expert is to provide input into the descriptive epidemiology of musculoskeletal conditions and to review the disease models and assumptions used in the estimation of the burden of disease. It is necessary to review the definitions and to define more specifically the natural history of the conditions and their evolution in different regions of the globe. It is also necessary to review the availability, quality and limitations of epidemiological data as a contribution to identifying alternative or new data sources, and to make recommendations for completing the picture, including extrapolating data from different populations. In this way it is possible to reach agreement on providing useful evidence in support of health policy and research.

3. Incidence and prevalence of musculoskeletal conditions

3.1 Introduction

A preliminary attempt has been made to identify sources of information on the incidence and prevalence of the five index conditions (rheumatoid arthritis, osteoarthritis, osteoporosis, spinal disorders and major limb traumas) for each WHO region (see Table 1). The results are given in the Annex. For each condition a literature search was conducted, and experts in musculoskeletal disorders from the respective regions were contacted. Maximal effort was used to obtain the raw data and present them broken down either into the age and gender bands used in the original survey or, where possible, into the age (see Section 2, page 12) and gender bands preferred by WHO. In those regions where more than one data source was available, data were selected which conformed to the preferred case definition outlined at the beginning of each section in the Annex. Where more than one survey used this case definition, the survey chosen was either the largest or the most representative of the region (either geographically or because it presented estimates which lay in the middle of the range obtained for the region). This issue rarely arose for regions other than Region of the Americas A and European Region A.

At this stage, no smoothing — e.g. weighted averaging of figures for adjacent age groups from surveys resulting in empty cells for certain age groups — was carried out to fill the empty cells. In some instances, however, the results of a number of small studies from the same region were combined. Those regions for which no data sets have so far been identified are highlighted, and suggestions are made as to where data might be obtained. An estimate derived from a different region is more likely to be correct than would be the assumption that a condition did not exist in a region with no data of its own. In some cases there are sufficient data from a region to indicate whether it is likely to be an area of high or low prevalence of a particular condition. There is, for example, limited information on the global epidemiology of osteoarthritis of the hip, yet regions seem to fall largely into either the high-prevalence or the low-prevalence category, few lying in the intermediate category. Even a small study may indicate in which of these two categories a region belongs with respect to the prevalence of osteoarthritis of the hip. An appropriate data set from a different region in the same prevalence category can then be used. The same process can be used to decide where further work is needed. It is not necessary for a comprehensive set of surveys to be conducted in every country. A few large surveys of high quality are needed from representative areas.

The eventual aim is to generate a set of tables for the incidence and prevalence of all the index conditions and for various subsets. There are currently insufficient data for some of these categories to permit any meaningful conclusions or comparisons, so tables are presented only for the prevalence of rheumatoid arthritis, osteoarthritis of the hip, osteoarthritis of the knee, generalized osteoarthritis, back pain (various definitions) and severe limb traumas, and for the incidence of fractured neck of femur.

3.1.1 *Potential further sources of data*

Because of the many gaps in the picture of the epidemiology of musculoskeletal disorders, the first priority is to identify existing sources of information that may have been missed. The most probable sources of currently missing data are papers published in languages other than English, and the grey literature, e.g. government-sponsored health surveys, national registries of physical disability and data on days lost from work through illness. Published studies do not always display the data in a format that can be used in the incidence and prevalence tables, so it is necessary to contact the researchers directly. In addition, not all the data collected in a survey may be included in a publication. For example, a survey on knee pain may also have yielded information on other pain which has never been fully analysed or published. Experts on musculoskeletal disorders who are working in particular countries or regions can most readily identify these data sources, and a network of such experts is being assembled.

3.1.2 *Recommendations for making estimates of incidence and prevalence of musculoskeletal conditions*

The task of compiling an accurate set of estimates of the number of individuals with musculoskeletal problems can never be completed. There will always be the possibility of a more up-to-date estimate or of focusing on a smaller geographical area or a more homogeneous population group. It is important to fill some of the major gaps, for example in Africa, South America, and Eastern Europe. Large surveys that investigate several conditions simultaneously are of more value than a series of small studies on single conditions. However, as estimating the number of cases of a condition is only the first step in making an assessment of health care needs, it may be necessary to move forward with rough estimates of numbers rather than delaying progress by waiting for precise figures. Other inflammatory arthropathies, such as gout and spondylarthropathies, and disabling pain syndromes that are not clearly defined also add to the global burden of musculoskeletal conditions. There are few estimates relating to these conditions, and future epidemiological studies should be aimed at overcoming this deficiency.

3.2 Rheumatoid arthritis

3.2.1 *Definition*

The definition of rheumatoid arthritis that is used in epidemiological studies has changed over time. The preferred definition now is that suggested by the American College of Rheumatology (ACR, Table 2) (*8*). The onset of rheumatoid arthritis should be considered to occur when a sufficient number of criteria are reached. There is no universal definition of childhood arthritis because of its less clear clinical pattern. The three common definitions are those developed by the ACR, the European League Against Rheumatism (EULAR) and, most recently, the International League of Associations for Rheumatology (ILAR) (*9*). They differ in nomenclature and have different inclusion and exclusion demands, each describing a somewhat distinct

Table 2
The 1987 revised criteria for the classification of rheumatoid arthritis (traditional format)[a]

Criterion	Definition
1. Morning stiffness	Morning stiffness in and around the joints, lasting at least one hour before maximal improvement
2. Arthritis of three or more joint areas	At least three joint areas simultaneously have had soft tissue swelling or fluid (not bony overgrowth alone) observed by a physician. The 14 possible areas are the right or left PIP, MCP, wrist, elbow, knee, ankle and MTP joints
3. Arthritis of hand joints	At least one area swollen (as defined above) in a wrist, MCP or PIP joint
4. Symmetrical arthritis	Simultaneous involvement of the same joint areas (as defined above) on both sides of the body (bilateral involvement of the PIPs, MCPs or MTPs is acceptable without absolute symmetry)
5. Rheumatoid nodules	Subcutaneous nodules, over bony prominences, or extensor surfaces, or in juxta-articular regions, observed by a physician
6. Serum rheumatoid factor	Demonstration of abnormal amounts of serum rheumatoid factor by any method for which the result has been positive in <5% of normal control subjects
7. Radiographic changes	Radiographic changes typical of rheumatoid arthritis on posteroanterior hand and wrist radiographs, which must include erosions or unequivocal bony decalcification localized in or most marked adjacent to the involved joints (osteoarthritic changes alone do not qualify)

PIP, proximal interphalangeal; MCP, metacarpophalangeal; MTP, metatarsophalangeal.
[a] For classification purposes, a patient shall be said to have rheumatoid arthritis if he/she has satisfied at least four of these seven criteria. Criteria one through four must have been present for at least six weeks. Patients with two clinical diagnoses are not excluded. Designation as classic, definite, or probable rheumatoid arthritis is *not* to be made.
Reproduced from reference *8*, with the permission of the publisher.

group of patients. The criteria of ILAR seek to describe homogeneous groups of patients in a manner that has been internationally agreed.

The direct interview and clinical examination of patients by a health professional or self-reporting could be used for the diagnosis of rheumatoid arthritis. A combination of these two approaches, such as self-administered screening questionnaires followed by the examination of positive responders, seems to work well in terms of sensitivity and economy. Longitudinal studies could be useful for defining diagnostic criteria; for this purpose, the area under the criteria curve could constitute an adequate measure. Other types of arthritis, such as reactive arthritis, gout, Lyme arthritis and others, should also be considered in terms of the global burden of disease. Conditions such as probable rheumatoid arthritis or undifferentiated arthritis, which could be prodromal stages of various arthropathies, should also be included in epidemiological studies but should be given a different weight to that of rheumatoid arthritis.

3.2.2 *Incidence*

Incidence data on rheumatoid arthritis have mostly been collected in populations of Anglo-Saxon ethnicity (*10*). The incidence of rheumatoid arthritis is 20–300 per 100000 subjects per year; that of juvenile rheumatoid arthritis is 20–50 per 100000 subjects per year (see Annex). Changes in the incidence and prevalence of rheumatoid arthritis are difficult to predict. Recent studies indicate a future decline in its incidence, particularly among women (*11*). On the other hand, its incidence is expected to increase over the next 10 years in Europe because of the increasing proportion of older people. The net result, however, is unpredictable, so prospective figures should be gathered in specific studies.

3.2.3 *Prevalence*

Data on the prevalence of rheumatoid arthritis derive largely from recently reviewed studies performed in the USA and Europe (*10*). The prevalence of rheumatoid arthritis in most industrialized countries varies between 0.3% and 1%, whereas in developing countries it is at the lower end of this range. Few cases or none were found in surveys in African populations (*12*) (see Annex). Because of the small number of patients identified, even in studies with large populations as the denominator, it is difficult to provide a complete picture of rheumatoid arthritis in any given area.

3.2.4 *Potential sources of further data*

Large numbers of additional data sets should be explored. The sources may be government surveys, insurance companies, health maintenance organizations, managed care organizations, government providers and pension fund records. Such sources are frequently underutilized in studies on musculoskeletal conditions because they are usually collected for different purposes. Data on different types of arthritis, such as infectious arthritis, gout and undifferentiated arthritis, which are more relevant in developing countries, should be also assimilated.

3.2.5 *Recommendations for making estimates of incidence and prevalence rates of the global burden*

There are two main reasons for the incompleteness of data on the incidence and prevalence of rheumatoid arthritis. First, data from

Africa, South America, and Asia are scant and need to be improved to allow an understanding of the intraregional and interregional variability of the disease. Second, several sets of data suggest that both the epidemiological and clinical features of rheumatoid arthritis vary over time. Repeat studies are therefore needed in particular areas in order to identify changing patterns of disease.

Epidemiological studies of rheumatoid arthritis in developing countries should have top priority. In areas where data are sparse, an extrapolation of incidence figures from neighbouring or similar countries could be used. However, this may be subject to social, economic, genetic and environmental variables, quite apart from issues of catchment area and rheumatoid arthritis definition. The need for rules to be used in the extrapolation and meta-analysis of data should be emphasized. This is a further area of research.

In addition there is a requirement to build databases of large cohorts of incident or prevalent patients to evaluate the changing presentation, clinical spectrum and different features of rheumatoid arthritis over time. Some such cohorts have already been studied in the United Kingdom (*13*) and other developed countries, but data from the developing countries are still lacking. This may be particularly important in specific situations, e.g. in rural areas that are becoming urbanized or in populations that have migrated to areas where the incidence of rheumatoid arthritis differs from that in the areas of origin.

3.3 Osteoarthritis

3.3.1 *Definition*

Osteoarthritis is not a simple disease entity and cannot be defined as such. However, a pathological concept binds together the different conditions covered by this term. The pathological definition is of a condition characterized by focal areas of loss of articular cartilage within the synovial joints, associated with hypertrophy of the bone (osteophytes and subchondral bone sclerosis) and thickening of the capsule. In this sense it is a reaction of the synovial joints to injury. This phenomenon can occur in any joint but is most common in certain joints of the hand, spine, knee, foot and hip.

This pathological change results, when severe, in radiological changes (loss of joint space, presence of osteophytes) that have been used in epidemiological studies to estimate the prevalence of osteoarthritis at different joint sites. A Lawrence, Bremner & Bier radiological osteoarthritis score of 2–4 is still the most widely used definition of radiological osteoarthritis in epidemiological studies (*14*).

Some people with these pathological (radiographic) changes have joint symptoms, i.e. pain, stiffness and loss of function, that are likely to be related to the presence of the joint pathology. These symptoms are not specific, and no clinical definition of osteoarthritis at any joint site has been properly validated. The symptoms vary with time, as well as between joint sites and individuals, and are dependent on many variables other than the joint damage (*15*). There are clinical criteria for the classification of osteoarthritis of hand, hip and knee (*16–18*), pain being an obligatory symptom in the osteoarthritis classification. However, these criteria have hardly been used in population studies because of the lack of validation.

3.3.2 *Incidence*

Because of the problems of definition the incidence of osteoarthritis cannot be estimated. The symptoms of osteoarthritis are not specific, and the radiological changes reflect a gradual pathological process for which no time of onset can be defined. An estimation of the incidence of severe osteoarthritis may be obtained from the figures of the progression of radiological osteoarthritis from a low to a higher Kellgren score, with or without the onset of clinical symptoms.

The Australian Burden of Disease and Injury Study (AUSBODI) (*19*) attempts to determine the incidence of osteoarthritis in Australia. As reliable incidence data for osteoarthritis are unavailable for the Australian population, the study has used the DISMOD software package to model incidence and duration from estimates of prevalence, remission, case-fatality rates and background mortality. Data derived from the DISMOD software indicate that females have a higher incidence of osteoarthritis than males in all age groups and that, overall, they have an incidence of 2.95 per 1000 population, compared with 1.71 per 1000 population in males. The estimated total incidences of osteoarthritis in Australia for males and females are 15 563 and 27 112 respectively. For women, the incidence of osteoarthritis is highest among those aged 65–74 years, reaching approximately 13.5 per 1000 population per year; for men, the highest incidence of approximately 9 cases per 1000 population per year occurs in those aged 75 years and over.

3.3.3 *Prevalence*

Most attempts to estimate the prevalence of osteoarthritis are based on radiographic surveys of populations. However, radiographs detect only cases of severe osteoarthritic pathology. They do not indicate whether patients have a problem (symptoms or disability). Radiographic surveys show that there is a strong age relationship with this pathology: osteoarthritic changes are uncommon in persons under the age of 40 but are seen in practically everyone over the age of 70 years (*20*).

There have been some attempts to estimate the number of people who might have significant clinical problems arising from osteoarthritic joint pathology. These have not been validated, but they suggest that about 10% of persons over the age of 60 are affected. Surveys have largely been conducted in the most developed countries, but there is indirect evidence suggesting that this is a worldwide problem. The Scientific Group estimates that 10% of the world's population who are 60 years or older have significant clinical problems that can be attributed to osteoarthritis.

In Australia the estimated total prevalence of osteoarthritis ranges from 6.4% in a 1995 national report (*21*) to 8.6% in the South Australian Health Omnibus Survey (ages ≥ 15 years) (*22*). The variability in prevalence reporting is caused by inherent variation between samples and by the use of different methods to ascertain the presence of osteoarthritis (self-reporting, diagnosis or modelling). The highest self-reported prevalence of osteoarthritis was measured in females ≥85 years of age bracket of the Health Omnibus Survey, for which a value of 57.1% was recorded. Australian prevalence studies show that females are more likely than males in all age brackets to have or self-report osteoarthritis.

AUSBODI has derived estimates of prevalence of osteoarthritis in Australia by means of the DISMOD software package, proposing a prevalence of 2.65% for males and 4.17% for females. AUSBODI has also estimated the prevalence of osteoarthritis in the country by age group and severity on the basis of radiologically defined criteria. It is important to note that osteoarthritis has not been radiologically defined for the Australian population and that the study has modelled prevalence, using data derived from a recent methodologically consistent study done in the Netherlands (*19*). The prevalences calculated from this section of the study range from 0.1% in the age group 25–34 years in both males and females to 26.93% in women aged ≥75 years.

3.3.4 *Potential sources of further data*

Large numbers of additional data sets should be explored, including government surveys and insurance company, health care and pension fund data, e.g. derived from health maintenance organizations, managed care organizations and government providers. These sources of information are frequently underutilized in studies on musculoskeletal conditions because they are usually collected for different purposes. However, they mainly contain data on self-reported diagnosis and symptoms, and comparison with population data based on radiological osteoarthritis classification is problematic. Consideration should be given to national osteoarthritis registries set up as periodic snapshots or longitudinal observation studies.

3.3.5 *Recommendations for making estimates of incidence and prevalence rates of the global burden*

The incidence and prevalence of musculoskeletal pain and disability in older people in all parts of the world should be considered as a matter of urgency. As outlined above, such pain and disability are extremely common and largely attributed to an ill-defined condition called osteoarthritis. The problem, however, is not what the disease is but its consequences and their determinants. The Global Burden of Disease Studies have made a welcome attempt to quantify the disease burden resulting from osteoarthritis, but there is a need for ongoing work so that the burden can be fully reflected.

The requirement for joint replacement surgery should also be addressed. Most joint replacements are carried out for people suffering from osteoarthritis, but rates per head of population and the severity of the condition at the time of surgery vary enormously between regions of the world, suggesting major inequities and a lack of clarity over who should have this intervention for advanced arthritis and when it should be undertaken.

3.4 Osteoporosis

3.4.1 *Definition*

Osteoporosis is defined as a systemic skeletal disease characterized by a low bone mass and a microarchitectural deterioration of bone tissue, with a consequent increase in bone fragility and susceptibility to fracture. In 1994 a WHO expert panel (*1*) operationalized this concept by defining diagnostic criteria for osteoporosis on the basis of measurement of bone mineral density (BMD).

- Osteoporosis: a BMD value more than 2.5 standard deviations below the mean BMD of young adult women (BMD T-score < –2.5).
- Osteopenia (low bone mass): a BMD value between 1 and 2.5 standard deviations below the mean BMD of young adult women (–2.5 < BMD T-score < –1).

Clinically, osteoporosis is recognized by the occurrence of characteristic low-trauma fractures, the best documented of these being hip, vertebral and distal forearm fractures.

Hip fracture

A hip fracture is a fracture of the proximal femur, either through the femoral neck (subcapital or transcervical fracture, an intracapsular fracture) or through the trochanteric region (intertrochanteric or subtrochanteric fracture, an extracapsular fracture). Intracapsular fractures are usually classified according to the Garden scale (*23*):

- — type I: incomplete;
- — type II: complete without displacement;
- — type III: complete with partial displacement;
- — type IV: complete with full displacement.

Extracapsular fractures are classified according to their stability (stable/unstable) and displacement (present/absent). These classification systems have a major influence on the choice of orthopaedic intervention, e.g. internal fixation or arthroplasty. Whether the etiology of the two fractures also differs remains contentious. Some studies, but not all, have suggested that osteoporosis plays a greater role in causing extracapsular fractures than it does in causing intracapsular fractures. The gold standard for fracture definition at the proximal femur is radiological.

Vertebral fracture

Vertebral fracture has been the most difficult osteoporosis-related fracture to define. The deformities that result from osteoporosis are usually classified into three categories:

- — crush (involving compression of the entire vertebral body);
- — wedge (in which there is anterior height loss);
- — biconcave (where there is a relative maintenance of the anterior and posterior heights, with central compression of the endplate regions).

The difficulty in deciding whether a vertebra is deformed arises from the variation in the shape of vertebral bodies both within the spine and between individuals. Initial studies of vertebral osteoporosis utilized subjective methods of defining the radiographic appearance of individual vertebral bodies. Such qualitative approaches often led to within-observer and between-observer disagreements over the presence or absence of deformity. This resulted in attempts to quantify deformity by using measurements of the vertebral dimensions. These morphometric approaches have culminated in algorithms comparing the extent to which ratios between the anterior-, posterior- and mid-vertebral heights (corresponding to wedge, biconcave and crush deformities) differ from vertebra-specific mean values in the general population. The normal ranges for these height ratios are estimated from a radiographic population survey, cut-off values for each type of deformity being arbitrarily assigned to points on the distribution of the ratios (3 or 4 standard deviations).

Although these morphometric approaches are widely utilized for research purposes, radiographic criteria for the semiquantitative assignment of vertebral deformities have also been derived. In the most extensively used system, vertebral deformities may be classified as mild (20–25% height loss), moderate (25–40% height loss) or severe (>40% height loss). In the northern USA, around one in three vertebral deformities reaches immediate clinical attention because of back pain, height loss or other functional impairment (*24*). Estimates of the proportion of vertebral deformities reaching primary care in Europe suggest that the figure here is lower, perhaps between 10% and 30% (*25*, *26*).

Distal forearm fracture

The most common distal forearm fracture is Colles fracture. This lies within 2.5 cm of the wrist joint margin and is associated with dorsal angulation and displacement of the distal fragment of the radius, often accompanied by a fracture of the ulnar styloid process. The reverse injury, known as Smith fracture, usually follows a forcible flexion injury to the wrist. It is relatively uncommon and tends to occur in young adults following major trauma. As with hip and vertebral fractures, distal forearm fractures require radiographic confirmation.

Rickets and osteomalacia

Although very different from osteoporosis, rickets and osteomalacia are also characterized by a low bone mineral content, and both may lead to bone pain and fractures. Rickets is characterized by a mineralization defect of newly formed bone in the growing skeleton. It leads to an increase in the amount of non-mineralized bone tissue (osteoid) and a thickening of growth plates. It causes bone pain, bone deformation, swelling of the joints and growth retardation (*27*). Osteomalacia is the adult counterpart of rickets and is characterized by an increase in osteoid tissue. Osteomalacia has been implicated in causing hip fracture in the elderly.

Rickets and osteomalacia are mainly attributable to a lack of exposure to sunlight because of climatic conditions, pollution that absorbs ultraviolet rays, clothing and the use of sunscreens. A low calcium intake aggravates the effects of vitamin D deficiency. Rare causes include congenital or acquired disorders of vitamin D metabolism, urinary phosphate loss, calcium deficiency, malabsorption syndromes

Table 3
Lifetime risk of fragility fractures in the Swedish population

Type of fracture	Lifetime risk at age 50 (%)	
	Women	Men
Hip	22.9	10.7
Distal forearm	20.8	4.6
Vertebral (clinical)	15.1	8.3
Proximal humerus	12.9	4.9
Any of the above	46.4	22.4

Source: reference *29*.

and an inhibition of mineralization by toxic substances such as fluoride and aluminium (*27*, *28*).

3.4.2 *Incidence*

The incidence of osteoporosis is best measured indirectly as the incidence of fractures resulting from the condition. The lifetime risk at the age of 50 years of fragility fractures is considerable (Table 3).

It is clear from the preceding section that estimates of the magnitude of osteoporosis and related fractures can be addressed in different ways. Incidence rates are best utilized to characterize the burden of fractures, whereas prevalence data may be applied to the frequency of reduced BMD or to the burden of vertebral deformities.

Hip fracture

In western populations the incidence of hip fractures increases exponentially with age. Above 50 years of age there is a female to male incidence ratio of approximately 2:1. Overall, about 98% of hip fractures occur among people aged 35 years and older, and 80% occur in women (because there are more elderly women than men) (*30*). Worldwide there were estimated to be 1.66 million hip fractures in 1990, about 1.19 million in women and 463000 in men (*31*, *32*). Most hip fractures occur after a fall from standing height or less in men or women with reduced bone strength. The risk of falling increases with age and is somewhat higher in elderly women than elderly men. There is some seasonality in the incidence of hip fractures: in temperate climates they tend to occur more frequently in the winter months than at other times. Most hip fractures, however, occur indoors rather than as a result of slipping on icy pavements.

These epidemiological characteristics apply principally to the incidence of hip fractures in Europe and the USA. However, data are now available from other parts of the world, including Africa, Latin America and China (including Hong Kong Special Administrative Region) (*32*). This information has been used to construct the incidence tables in the Annex. Hip fracture generally occurs less frequently in non-Caucasian than in Caucasian populations. Incidence rates are extremely low in African countries and greater among South-East Asian populations. The highest incidence rates have been reported from northern Europe and the northern part of the USA. Even within a given ethnic group there is considerable variation in the incidence of hip fracture. Thus, rates vary by a factor of about 10 between Sweden and Turkey. These variations imply an important role for environmental factors in the incidence of hip fracture. The observation that differences in incidence between countries are much larger than those between Caucasian women and Caucasian men suggests that factors other than estrogen deficiency are significant (*33*).

Patients with hip fractures in developed countries are hospitalized, so the total number of cases is easy to determine. In rural areas of other countries, however, patients may not be hospitalized and may be treated at home, making an assessment for the entire world problematic. Most studies in Asia have been performed in major cities. Better estimates are needed for large parts of the world, but data for small areas in these parts can currently be used.

A working group of the International Osteoporosis Foundation has commenced a study on the incidence of hip fracture by examining national registration systems throughout the world. This supplements WHO initiatives aiming to characterize the global burden of osteoporosis.

Vertebral fracture

Incidence rates for morphometric vertebral deformities have been obtained from the European Prospective Osteoporosis Study. As part of this study, lateral thoracolumbar X-rays were obtained under standardized conditions from a sample of 15570 men and women aged 50–79 years who were enrolled from population registers in 19 European countries. The incidence of new vertebral deformities was estimated from X-rays at baseline and at four-year follow-up. Overall, age-adjusted and sex-adjusted incidence rates for vertebral deformity were 1% per year among women and 0.6% per year among men (*34*).

Similar incidence estimates have been reported from the Framingham Study and from the Study of Osteoporotic Fractures in the USA, where spinal X-rays have been obtained for some 8000 women. Other sources of incidence data for vertebral deformities have included the Rotterdam Study and a study in Hiroshima, Japan (*35*). There are no data from Africa or South America.

The age-adjusted incidence of clinically diagnosed vertebral fractures has been estimated in the northern part of the USA. For Caucasian women aged 50 years and over it was estimated to be 5.3 per thousand person-years, the comparable male rate being around half this figure (*36*). Among men the incidence rate climbs exponentially with age, adopting a pattern similar to that observed for hip fractures in the same population. Among women there is a more linear increase in incidence with age, such that the vertebral fracture rate is higher than that for hip fracture before the age of 70 years but not thereafter (*34*). Falls account for only one-third of new vertebral fractures among men and women in the USA. The majority of such fractures are the result of compressive loading associated with other activities such as lifting or changing positions, or have been discovered only incidentally. Whereas 90% of clinically diagnosed vertebral fractures in women occurred as a result of moderate or minimal trauma in this study, a substantial proportion (37%) of those among men occurred as a result of severe trauma.

The final means of studying the incidence of vertebral fractures is to confine rates to those of hospitalized subjects, for whom data can be obtained from national registers. Such a register-based study in Europe (*37*) suggested an incidence rate of hospitalized vertebral fracture that is substantially smaller than the estimates of all vertebral fractures coming to clinical attention (perhaps 1–2% of all incident vertebral deformities). This result is not surprising, because most people with vertebral fractures are not hospitalized. In this European study, however, there was a striking geographical correlation between the incidence of hospitalized vertebral fracture cases and that of hip fracture cases among different countries.

Distal forearm fracture

Distal forearm fractures display a different pattern of incidence from those of hip and vertebral fractures. Incidence studies in the northern USA in the early 1990s suggested that the rate increased linearly among women between the ages of 40 and 65 years, thereafter appearing to level off. Among men, the incidence rate remained constant between the ages of 20 and 80 years (*36*, *38*). Thus most distal forearm fractures occur in women (the age-adjusted female to male ratio being 4:1), and around 50% occur in women aged 65 years and older. The reason for the previously observed plateau in the incidence rate among females above the age of 65 years remains unknown, but it has been suggested that it reflects a change in the pattern of falls with advancing age as a consequence of loss of neuromuscular protective reflexes.

A more recent multicentre study in the United Kingdom found annual incidences of 9 and 37 per 10000 men and women respectively, with hospitalization rates of 23% and 19% respectively (*39*). There was a tendency for the incidence rate of distal forearm fracture to continue to increase after the age of 70 years among women, perhaps pointing to increasing frailty in the elderly female population of developed countries throughout the last decade of the twentieth century and the first decade of the twenty-first.

All fractures

The majority of fractures in subjects aged over 50 years are the result of osteoporosis. Epidemiological studies of these age-related fractures have been performed in Australia, Sweden, the United Kingdom and the northern USA. The incidence rates of proximal humeral, pelvic and proximal tibial fractures rise steeply with age and are greater in women than in men. About 80% of proximal humeral fractures occur in individuals aged 35 years and over, three-quarters occurring in women (*40*). The same general picture is seen in populations of other developed countries. Similar patterns have been observed for distal femur fracture and fractures of the rib, clavicle and scapula.

Not all fractures, even those occurring in persons over the age of 50 years, are the result of osteoporosis. Attempts to classify fracture have varied. Some have involved the use of expert opinion to indicate that a fixed proportion of fractures at a specific site are caused by osteoporosis. Others classify osteoporotic fractures as the result of low energy or low bone mass. None of these classifications is, however, ideal. There does appear to be a constant relationship between hip fracture burden and the burden caused by fractures at other sites. Since the hip fracture rate is known in many regions of the world, a methodology has been devised to calculate the osteoporosis fracture burden from the hip fracture rate (*40*).

3.4.3 *Prevalence*

Bone mineral density

Implicit in the definition of osteoporosis using BMD alone is the notion of a relationship between this parameter and fracture risk. A low BMD is therefore analogous to high blood pressure or an elevated serum cholesterol concentration. The risk of fracture rises when BMD declines, just as the risk of stroke rises with blood pressure and hypercholesterolaemia leads to an increased risk of myocardial infarction. WHO operationalized this concept by considering osteoporosis to be present when the BMD level in women was more than 2.5 standard deviations below the normal mean for young women. In order to provide some comparability with definitions that incorporated fracture, the subset of women with presumptive osteoporosis who also had a history of one or more fragility fractures were deemed to have severe or established osteoporosis.

Many sites of the skeleton are accessible for BMD measurement. Moreover, there are many measurement techniques, so that there are no standardized criteria on the prevalence of osteoporosis on a multinational basis. Specific data on the prevalence of osteoporosis as defined by WHO have been obtained in Australian, European and North American populations. In the northern USA it is estimated that 54% of postmenopausal Caucasian women have osteopenia, and a further 30% have osteoporosis in at least one skeletal site. Furthermore, it is estimated that osteoporosis is established (BMD more than 2.5 standard deviations below the normal mean for young women, and a history of low-trauma fracture) in 51% of osteoporotic women and in 16% of all Caucasian women aged 50 years or above. In the United Kingdom, it is estimated that around 23% of women aged 50 years or more have osteoporosis as defined by WHO. The proportion increases steeply between the ages of 50 and 80 years. The prevalences of osteoporosis, as defined by WHO, in relation to age in Sweden and the USA are indicated in Tables 4 and 5.

The International Osteoporosis Foundation has recently recommended that, for the purposes of diagnosis as opposed to those of assessment, BMD should be measured at the hip using dual-energy X-ray absorptiometry (DXA). It is also recommended that a referent standard derived from the USA population be used (*42*). On the basis of these criteria the general prevalence of osteoporosis rises from 5%

Table 4
Percentages of Swedish women with osteoporosis[a]

Age range (years)	Osteoporosis of the hip alone (%)
50–59	7.0
60–69	22.0
70–79	31.0
80–89	36.0

[a] Defined as a bone mineral density more than 2.5 standard deviations below the young adult reference mean at the hip.
Reproduced from reference *41* with permission of the publisher.

Table 5
Percentage of Caucasian women with osteoporosis[a] (adjusted to 1990 Caucasian women in the USA)

Age range in years	Osteoporosis at any site (%)	Osteoporosis of the hip alone (%)
30–39	0	0
40–49	0	0
50–59	14.8	3.9
60–69	21.6	8.0
70–79	38.5	24.5
80+	70.0	47.5
≥50	30.3	16.2

[a] Defined as a bone mineral density more than 2.5 standard deviations below the young adult reference mean at the spine, hip or mid-radius.
Source: reference *1*.

in women at the age of 50 years to 50% at the age of 85, the comparable figures in men being 2.4% and 20% (*43*). It is noteworthy that among the countries studied to date the prevalence of osteoporosis according to criteria based on BMD varies far less than does fracture incidence. Data from the Lebanese reference population are, for example, similar to the above data from Sweden and the USA. Further studies of the global burden of osteoporosis should include estimates of the prevalence of the disorder using BMD based criteria in other parts of the world.

Rickets and osteomalacia

Rickets is relatively rare in developed countries but still occurs as a consequence of dietary deficiency (a macrobiotic diet) or wearing too much clothing (*44*). In Ethiopia, low serum concentrations of 25-hydroxyvitamin D have been reported (*45*), and rickets caused by calcium deficiency has been encountered in Central Africa (*46*). Osteomalacia may also occur in countries at low latitudes where there is abundant sunshine, especially when extensive clothing prevents skin exposure. Low serum concentrations of 25-hydroxyvitamin D in adults and the elderly have been reported from Italy and the Eastern Mediterranean (*47*, *48*).

In Europe and the USA, osteomalacia mainly occurs in the elderly as a result of a lack of exposure to sunshine which is not compensated by adequate vitamin D intake (*44*). It is estimated that 1–5% of hip fractures in the elderly are caused by osteomalacia (*49*). A less severe degree of vitamin D deficiency causes secondary hyperparathyroidism and cortical bone loss, which also may lead to fractures (*50*). Osteomalacia is fairly common in people from India and the Eastern Mediterranean who have emigrated to Western Europe.

Osteomalacia can easily be cured by dietary supplementation with vitamin D and calcium, but more data are needed on the prevalence of the condition in order to develop adequate prevention programmes.

3.4.4 *Potential sources of further data*

On an international basis the risk of hip fracture varies much more than can be explained on the basis of BMD alone. This limits the value of estimates of the prevalence of osteoporosis. Factors other than BMD contribute independently to the risk of fracture; they include age, a prior fragility fracture, a family history of fracture, a low body mass index (BMI), immobility, smoking and excessive alcohol consumption. Collectively, these risk factors are quantitatively more important than BMD. For this reason, estimates of the future burden of osteoporosis would be better characterized as probabilities of osteoporotic fracture. The assessment of such probabilities depends on a knowledge of internationally validated risk factors and a more detailed knowledge of fracture incidence than is currently available. Hip fracture rates are known for fewer than 40 countries, and even less information is available for other types of fracture. A substantial investment in epidemiological research is therefore required.

3.4.5 *Recommendations for making estimates of incidence and prevalence rates of the global burden*

There are no internationally derived data on the incidence and prevalence of osteoporosis based on BMD as defined by WHO. However, the utility of providing this information is not high. Efforts should therefore be directed towards an accurate documentation of the incidence of osteoporotic fractures in different countries. It is recommended that countries provide the mechanisms whereby hospitalized fractures in the elderly can be documented. Where possible, registers should be provided of osteoporotic fractures that are not commonly hospitalized (e.g. vertebral fractures and fractures of the distal forearm and proximal humerus).

- Further information is required on the global variation in the incidence of hip, vertebral, distal forearm and other fractures. Incidence estimates for vertebral and distal forearm and other limb fractures are scanty, especially in Asian populations and in Africa and Latin America.
- Information on the prevalence of osteopenia and osteoporosis, based on densitometric criteria, is required for Africa, Asia and Latin America.

- Data on hospital admission for vertebral, forearm and other limb fractures should be collected.
- There is an urgent need for studies on the prevalence of rickets and osteomalacia in Africa and Asia as these diseases can be easily cured by vitamin D and/or calcium supplementation.

3.5 Spinal disorders

3.5.1 *Definition*

Spinal disorders are a wide and heterogeneous range of specific diseases and nonspecific musculoskeletal disorders involving the spinal column (Table 6). Specific diseases of the spine include trauma, mechanical injury, spinal cord injury, inflammation, infection and tumour. Nonspecific musculoskeletal disorders of the spine include maladies affecting the muscles, nerves, intervertebral discs, joints, cartilage, tendons and ligaments of the neck and back. Complaints about pain involving the neck and back are the primary manifestation of most spinal disorders. The incidence of spinal disorders varies with age, most conditions being distributed throughout the life span (Figure 3).

Specific causes

The specific etiologies of spinal disorders are classified as traumatic, congenital, inflammatory, infectious, metabolic and malignant. Acute spinal disorders resulting from traumas are most often fractures causing spinal cord injury, dislocation and spinal dysfunction. Chronic spinal disorders resulting from repetitive intervertebral disc traumas are frequently caused by a focal extension of the disc beyond the vertebral end-plate, producing radicular symptoms attributable to nerve compromise.

Spinal infection may result from vertebral osteomyelitis (pyogenic, granulomatous or other infectious processes), epidural abscess or inflammation of the intervertebral disc. Although these spinal disorders are rare in most countries, both mortality and morbidity are significant if appropriate treatment is not instigated. Congenital abnormalities include spondylolisthesis, spina bifida, scoliosis and other malformations. Spinal disorders may be the result of metabolic disease processes, including osteoarthritis, osteoporosis, osteomalacia and osteitis deformans. Spinal disorders resulting from tumour include metastases, primary malignant tumours (chordoma and myeloma) and benign tumours (osteoid ostema, osteoblastoma and osteochrondroma). Inflammatory diseases affecting the spine include rheumatoid arthritis, ankylosing spondylitis, Reiter syndrome and psoriatic arthritis.

Table 6
Classification of spinal disorders

Specific (15–20%)

- Congenital
  - Interspinous pseudarthrosis
  - Scoliosis
  - Spina bifida
  - Spondylolisthesis
  - Vertebral epiphysitis
- Degenerative
  - Spinal stenosis
  - Spondylolisthesis
- Infectious
  - Epidural abscess
  - Osteomyelitis
    - Bacterial
    - Tuberculosis (Pott disease)
    - Other infections
  - Paraspinous abscess
  - Septic arthritis
  - Septic discitis
- Inflammatory
  - Arthritides
    - Ankylosing spondylitis
    - Juvenile rheumatoid arthritis
    - Psoriatic spondylitis (sacroiliitis)
    - Reiter syndrome
    - Rheumatoid arthritis
    - Seronegative spondyloarthropathy
  - Fibrosis secondary to inflammation
    - Arachnoiditis
    - Epineural fibrosis
    - Intraneural fibrosis
  - Inflammation of nerve roots
    - Neuritis
    - Radiculitis
  - Vertebral osteochondritis
- Metabolic
  - Osteochondrosis (Scheuerman disease)
  - Osteomalacia
  - Osteopenia
  - Osteoporosis
  - Osteitis fibrocystica
  - Ochronotic spondylosis
  - Paget disease
- Neoplastic
  - Bone tumour
    - Benign
    - Malignant
    - Metastatic
  - Intradural and epidural tumours
  - Meningeal carcinomatosis
  - Multiple myeloma
- Traumatic
  - Dislocation or subluxation
  - Fractures of the vertebrae
  - Intervertebral disc herniation

Nonspecific (80–85%)

- Degenerative
  - Degenerative disc
  - Degenerative joint
  - Facet joint
  - Herniated intervertebral disc
  - Hyperlordosis
  - Kyphosis
  - Lumbar spondylosis
  - Osteoarthritis
  - Osteophytes
  - Spinal instability
- Idiopathic back pain
- Muscular disorders
  - Acute muscle fatigue
  - Acute strain
  - Acute reflex muscle spasm
  - Chronic strain
  - Fibromyalgia
  - Myofascial pain syndrome
- Traumatic
  - Apophyseal (facet) joint disorder
  - Coccydynia
  - Episacral lipoma
  - Intervertebral disc herniation
  - Lumbosacral joint sprain
  - Muscle atrophy
  - Postural disorders
  - Sacroiliac joint sprain
  - Whiplash

Referred back pain

- Congenital
  - Sickle-cell anaemia
- Neoplastic
  - Lymphoma
- Infectious
  - Abdominal abscess
  - Bacterial endocarditis
- Retroperitoneal masses
  - Carcinomatous lymphadenopathy
  - Lymphosarcoma

Table 6 *(Continued)*

Hodgkin's disease	Visceral
Vascular	Kidney or ureter
Aortic aneurysm	Stomach and colon
Embolism of the renal artery	Urinary bladder and prostate
Myocardial ischaemia	Uterus and adnexa
Myocardial infarction	

Nonspecific causes

Musculoskeletal disorders of the spine are classified as nonspecific if no underlying disease (e.g. ankylosing spondylitis), pathophysiological mechanism (e.g. trauma or malignancy) or anatomical source of pain (e.g. facet joint, disc herniation, muscle or nerve root) is identified by simple clinical means such as clinical examination, radiological studies and basic laboratory tests. Nonspecific musculoskeletal conditions are by far the most frequent causes of spinal disorders and have the greatest impact on individuals, health care systems and societies as a whole.

It is worth noting that, even after extensive evaluation, only 15% of patients presenting with acute low back problems can be given a definitive diagnosis (*52*). Nonspecific musculoskeletal spinal disorders are often reported as low back pain. Such pain of less than seven days' duration is not a disease but a complaint that can turn into a complex syndrome. Unfortunately, the literature abounds with studies confusing the prevalence of the symptom of low back pain with the incidence of spinal disorders, partly because of the lack of standardization and validation of the terminology and classification of spinal disorders. These factors account for some of the heterogeneity, differences and contradictory findings in the literature regarding diagnosis, epidemiology, treatment and rehabilitation (*53*, *54*). This lack of standardization and validation of terminology and classification imposes a significant limitation on the use of epidemiological data of spinal disorders.

Nonspecific spinal disorders are classified as acute (duration less than one month) or subacute (duration up to three months) if they occur suddenly after a prolonged period (six months) without pain and with a retrospective duration of less than three months. These disorders are categorized as chronic if they occur episodically within a six-month period or last for more than three months. They are usually accompanied by other musculoskeletal pains, bodily complaints, psychological distress and, often in chronic cases, amplified dysfunctional cognition and pain behaviour. The etiology of nonspecific spinal

Figure 3
Age at peak incidence of selected spinal disorders[a]

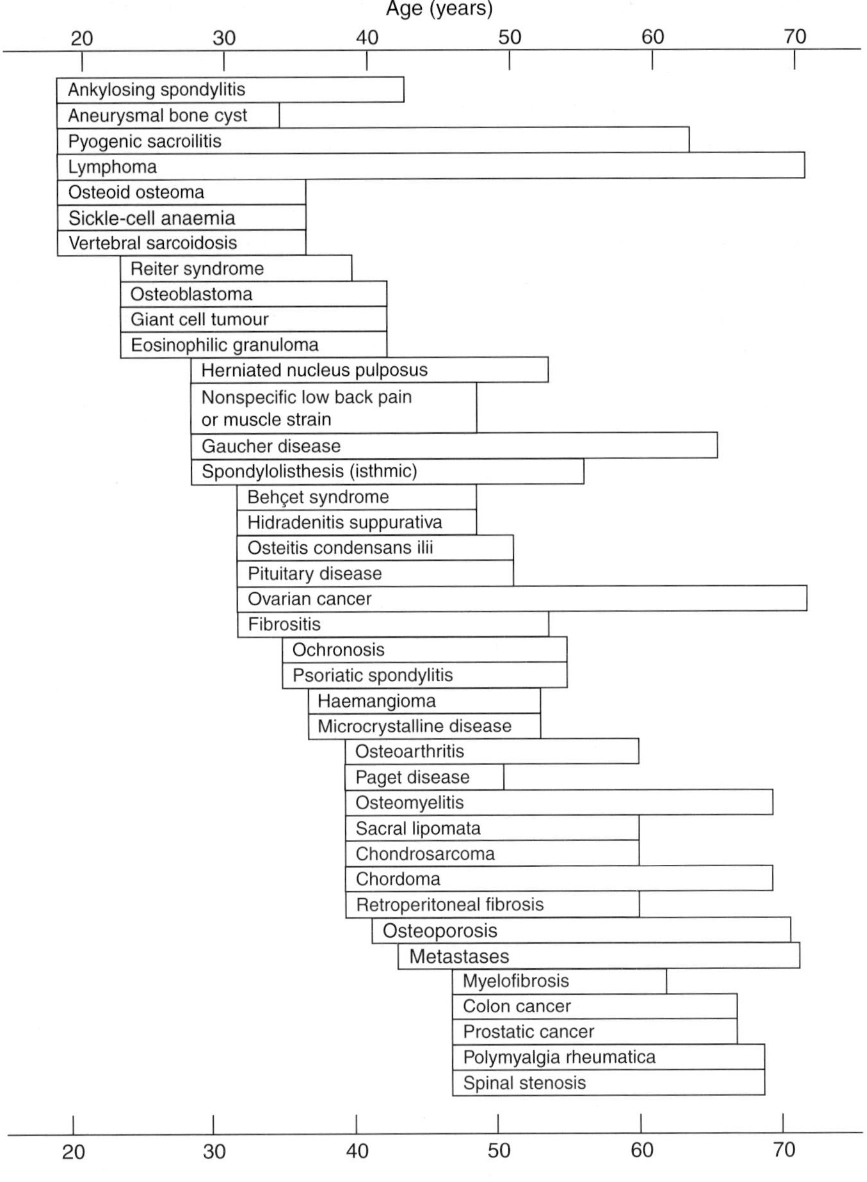

[a] Modified from reference *51* with permission of the publisher.

WHO 03.104

disorders is generally difficult to ascertain because of the long history and low specificity of physical signs and symptoms.

Nonspecific spinal disorders manifest a wide spectrum of actual severity, but there is often a discrepancy between the reported level of pain and loss of function on the one hand and the observed minimal physical signs on the other. Of the numerous pathological conditions of the spine reported worldwide, nonspecific spinal disorders in the cervical, thoracic and lumbar regions comprise the vast majority of problems found in workers. Because of the lack of a uniform and comprehensive method of gathering and tracking data on nonspecific spinal disorders, a coordinated and standardized system of data collection is needed. There is a need to build databases on large cohorts of people in order to evaluate the incidence, prevalence, clinical spectrum and features of spinal disorders over time. Standardized coding procedures as well as more precise and consistent descriptions of risk factors should also be developed for these large data systems.

Numerous studies on the epidemiology of spinal disorders have been published over the past 60 years. In general their results are hard to compare and summarize because of the profound methodological heterogeneity of the studies (e.g. in relation to sampling frames and procedures, the formulation of questions, interview techniques, instruments, the wording of questions, the characterization of pain, non-response bias, the region of the back, the point in time and the duration of pain). The two following observations can, however, be made.

1. There has been no apparent increase in the prevalence of nonspecific spinal disorders over the past 30 years, although the number of relevant studies is small and geographically limited. However, the problem is becoming more widely recognized, especially in developed countries, as the impact of cost and morbidity is more extensively reported in the medical and lay press.
2. There are clear indications of an increase in disability associated with spinal disorders being reported in connection with social security in many countries. It is therefore useful to distinguish the incidence and prevalence of spinal complaints and disorders from the observation of disability related to spinal disorders. The increase in social security disability arising from spinal disorders may be attributable to an ageing population, improved disability benefits or both. It is also possible that culture-specific factors have affected the awareness and reporting of symptoms.

3.5.2 *Incidence*

Population-based incidence data on spinal disorders have been collected primarily in North America and Europe (*53*, *55*, *56*). No extrapolation to other ethnic groups and geographical areas has been attempted because of the limited data available. These data may be subject to social, economic, genetic and environmental variables, in addition to issues of study technique and spinal disorder definition. A meta-analysis of the existing data could be useful, but the methods and criteria used in different studies are a major source of concern. Rules for data sets on spinal disorders should be developed in order to overcome this problem for future meta-analyses.

Specific causes

The incidence of these disorders in most industrialized countries varies between 1% and 10%. In developing countries the incidence is at the lower end of this range (see Annex). Unfortunately, epidemiological data on many spinal disorders with specific causes and all spinal disorders with nonspecific causes are often reported as relating to low back pain regardless of the diagnosis or cause. In many studies, this heterogeneity is less than defining for functional limiting disease processes.

Nonspecific causes

The incidence of these disorders in most industrialized countries varies between 4% and 5% annually (*53, 55–57*). These data are reported in the Annex. It is difficult to define and identify the more significant and severe episodes since their relevance (e.g. as a starting point of chronification) may be assessed only retrospectively. Retrospective reports of back pain characteristics are notoriously unreliable because the past occurrences of diseases and symptoms are usually underreported in questionnaire surveys.

The traditional epidemiological concept of incidence is also difficult to apply to the experience of back pain because of its unstable, episodic nature and the uncertainty of onset of any episode. Although the spontaneous recovery in a single episode suggests that nonspecific spinal disorders are self-limiting disease processes, recent studies provide evidence of a fluctuating, recurrent and intermittent course of nonspecific musculoskeletal spinal disorders in adults which may lead to a chronic phase (*58, 59*).

Mortality data are of limited relevance for nonspecific musculoskeletal spinal disorders. In addition, the reporting of a given episode or condition seems to depend on the system of social security, national health care and worker compensation in the country concerned. The information obtained is significantly influenced by differences between societies and individuals. Data derived from workers' compensation claims are administrative records that provide comprehensive records of wages lost, treatment costs and time off work. However, these records do not include all data because of limited coverage of the total workforce, incomplete or no reporting, inaccurate diagnosis or a failure to indicate degrees of severity.

3.5.3 *Prevalence*

Some cohorts have already been studied in the USA (*60–62*; American Academy of Orthopaedic Surgeons, personal communication, 2000) and western Europe (*63–66*). A small amount of information has been reported from other parts of the world (*67*), and these studies have been reviewed (*68–71*). The trends recognized in these studies may be particularly important in specific situations, for instance in rural areas that are becoming urbanized or in migrant populations moving to areas where the incidence of spinal disorders differs from that in the areas of origin.

Mortality and comorbidity in these cohorts are also relevant. A decline in the lifetime occurrence of low back pain in the highest age category has been noted in several surveys. Possible explanations for this include limited recall of past events, an altered perception or reporting of current episodes, selective mortality or a cohort effect (i.e. individuals now over the age of 65 years may, for unknown reasons, have a lower likelihood of low back pain throughout their lives). Some data suggest selective mortality exists among patients with nonspecific musculoskeletal spinal disorders, possibly because of associated health habits or socioeconomic circumstances (*60*). The mechanisms of interaction between spinal disorders and other diseases that may affect the same patients are largely unknown. This information, as well as data on the interaction between spinal disorders and the treatment of comorbid conditions, should be evaluated.

Specific causes

The prevalence of these diseases in most industrialized countries varies between 2% and 8%; in developing countries it is at the lower end of this range (see Annex).

Nonspecific causes

Most of the available data on the prevalence of nonspecific musculoskeletal spinal disorders were obtained from studies performed in the USA and Europe, and have been reviewed (*63*, *68*, *70*, *71*). The lifetime prevalence of these disorders in most industrialized countries varies between 60% and 85%; in developing countries it is at the lower end of this range (see Annex).

3.5.4 *Potential sources of further data*

Additional existing data sets should be evaluated as data sources. These may include data obtained from government surveys, health maintenance organizations, managed care organizations and government providers. These sources of information are frequently underutilized in studies on musculoskeletal conditions because they are usually collected for different purposes.

3.5.5 *Recommendations for making estimates of incidence and prevalence rates of the global burden*

A uniform epidemiological data set is required in order to facilitate comparative research and to render results comparable. The epidemiology of spinal disorders in the lumbar spine has been extensively studied in most developed countries, but the data from Eastern Europe and the rest of the world are limited (*68*, *70*, *71*). Information relating to populations and health care in developing countries is urgently needed. Prospective figures should be gathered through specific studies. New studies should use uniform classification and include data on disability and comorbity in spinal disorders. Epidemiological studies of spinal disorders in developing countries should be given high priority. Rules governing the extrapolation and meta-analysis of the existing data should be laid down. The extrapolation of data may be influenced by social, economic, genetic and environmental variables, as well as study techniques and definitions of spinal disorders. Extrapolation should be performed with caution, and guidelines on the process should be developed in pilot studies so that conclusions can be drawn with respect to areas where data are not available or epidemiological studies are not feasible. A meta-analysis of existing data could be useful, but the methods and criteria used in different studies are a major source of concern. Rules for data sets on spinal disorder should be developed so as to overcome this problem for future meta-analysis.

3.6 Severe limb trauma

3.6.1 *Definition*

The Working Group on Limb Trauma adopted the following operational definition. Major limb traumas are all acute injuries and burns affecting the upper and lower extremities, excluding sprains, strains and superficial injuries such as minor lacerations and contusions. This definition includes all fractures, dislocations, crushing injuries, open wounds, amputations, burns and neurovascular injuries to the extremities. Injuries resulting from all mechanisms (including both intentional and unintentional injuries) are included in the definition.

Table 7
Nature of limb traumas[a]: codes of the International Classification of Diseases

	Upper extremity	Lower extremity
Fractures	810–819	808, 820–829
Crushing injuries	927	928
Dislocations	831–834	835–838
Open wounds	880–884	890–894
Amputations	885–887	895–897
Burns	943–944	945
Blood vessels	903	904
Nerve injuries	955	956

[a] Excluded from the definition are sprains and strains (840–846, 848.5), superficial injuries/ contusions (912–917, 923–924) and other/unspecified (959.2–959.5, 959.6–959.7).

Lower extremity traumas (LET) include injuries to the pelvis (and distal regions). Upper extremity traumas (UET) include all injuries to the shoulder (and distal areas). Table 7 provides the corresponding codes used in the International Classification of Diseases (ICD) for each category of LET and UET.

Some concern was expressed that this definition might be too inclusive, encompassing injuries that typically do not require medical attention and/or result in very limited or no impairment or disability. The exclusion of sprains and strains, together with contusions and minor lacerations, leaves out many but not all of these minor injuries. However, it was recognized that some sprains and strains (e.g. acute neck strain) might result in significant disability and would not be covered by the definition as currently constructed. It was also noted that specific musculoskeletal injuries were excluded from the definition and did not appear to belong to any of the other groups of conditions currently defined by the Bone and Joint Decade monitoring project. Most notably, cumulative trauma disorders are not included in the definition of major limb traumas.

3.6.2 *Incidence*

Principal sources of data on the incidence or occurrence of major limb trauma include:

— administrative databases or registries maintained by health care providers (e.g. hospitals, clinics and emergency departments);
— administrative databases maintained by insurers or payers of health care (e.g. workers' compensation schemes, government assistance programmes and private insurance companies);
— community health surveys that ask people to recall injury events within a given period;

— special databases constructed to monitor the incidence of specific types or mechanisms of injury (e.g. assaults, injuries associated with motor vehicles, work-related injuries).

Data maintained by health care facilities are usually available in both developing countries and established market economies. They also provide more reliable information on the nature of injury than do surveys based on self-reporting. They may, however, lead to significant underestimation of the true incidence of limb traumas if access to health care is not equitable at all levels of the health system.

Data on the incidence of major limb traumas were presented from selected countries and are summarized below. In the USA there are several sources of data on this subject. The National Health Interview Survey (NHIS) provides one of the more comprehensive estimates of the number of all injuries that occur among the civilian, non-institutionalized population (*72*). Included in the NHIS definition are all injuries that are either medically attended or result in one or more days of restricted activity. Incidence rates based on these NHIS data are presented in the Annex (these figures exclude pelvic fractures, burns and isolated neurovascular injuries). In 1996 there were 17895000 reported limb injuries, a rate of 67.7 per 1000 population. The rates for lower and upper limb traumas were 41.2 and 26.5 per 1000 persons respectively. The highest rates occurred in the age groups 5–34 and ≥76 years.

Also in the USA, the Healthcare Cost and Utilization Project Nationwide Inpatient Sample (HCUP-NIS) provides estimates of the number of limb injuries resulting in a hospital stay of one or more nights (*73*). These data provide estimates of the incidence of more severe limb traumas, as defined by the need for hospitalization within the context of the United States health care system. For the purpose of this report, only discharges with a first-listed diagnosis of limb trauma were counted. In 1996, limb traumas (LET and UET combined) accounted for 930435 hospital discharges, a rate of 3.5 per 1000 population. Limb injuries constitute the leading cause of all trauma admissions in the USA, accounting for approximately half the total. Hospitalizations for lower limb injuries occur at a rate of 2.7 per 1000, those for upper limb injuries at a rate of 0.8 per 1000. These rates are summarized by age and gender in the Annex. In the USA and other established market economies, approximately half the injuries to extremities which result in hospitalization are attributable to falls. Road traffic accidents account for an additional 15–20%. Approximately 20% of the instances of hospitalization associated with injuries to the upper extremities are attributable to machinery and tools.

Data similar to those described above are available from other countries in the Americas and from Australia, Europe, Israel and New Zealand. The published reports available to the working group were not, however, sufficiently detailed to allow the derivation of estimates of incidence as defined above. Injury statistics are more typically reported by mechanism (e.g. road traffic accidents, falls, assaults, etc.) than by the specific nature of the injuries (e.g. fracture, open wound, crush injury) or the affected region(s) of the body. Differences in the definition of limb trauma also make it difficult to compare data between countries. Some figures include sprains and strains, whereas others exclude these relatively minor injuries. In many instances, only overall estimates of orthopaedic injuries, typically including back injuries and, in some cases, cumulative trauma disorders, are reported.

Data from Africa and Asia are generally less readily available. Household survey data were presented from two areas in Ghana, one urban (Kumasi) and one rural (Brong-Ahafo) (*74*). The survey gathered data on acute injuries occurring during the preceding year and included only those resulting in a loss of one or more days of normal activity. From these data the incidence rates of severe limb injury were estimated. A severe limb injury was defined as one resulting in 30 or more days of disability. Such injuries were estimated to occur at a rate of 17.0 per 1000 persons per year, the values for the rural and urban areas being 22.1 and 12.9 per 1000 respectively. It should be noted that only injuries caused by blunt and penetrating mechanisms were included. Injuries caused by burns and snakebites were excluded; had they been included, the rates would have been approximately 10% higher. The rates are given by age and gender in the Annex.

Preliminary estimates of the global incidence of limb trauma in the USA were developed for the two major causes, i.e. falls and road traffic accidents, which account for nearly three-quarters of limb injuries that result in hospitalization. These estimates were derived by multiplying the age-specific and gender-specific estimates of falls and motor vehicle injuries (*75*) by the corresponding estimates of the proportions of hospitalizations with a first-listed diagnosis of limb injury. The latter estimates were obtained from the United States HCUP-NIS hospitalization data as described above. For all ages and both genders the proportions of hospitalizations resulting from major limb traumas were 0.82 and 0.42 for falls and road traffic accidents respectively. Although these figures are likely to vary somewhat between regions of the world, they provide some indication of what to expect in the presence of a certain incidence of falls and road traffic accidents. The resulting estimates for each WHO region are given in the Annex.

3.6.3 *Prevalence*

The prevalence of limb traumas is difficult to define in the traditional sense because injuries are acute events that have no duration per se. One approach is to define it by its consequences. Thus the prevalence of limb traumas could be defined as the number of people living in a population at a specific time with a loss, deformity or impairment of a limb that has been caused by trauma.

Estimates of the number of people living with the consequences of limb trauma were presented for Ghana and the USA. The United States estimates are based on the NHIS and include all persons who report living with the loss, deformity or impairment of a limb as the result of an injury. In 1996 this number was estimated to be 9475875 (35.8 per 1000 people), representing 12% of all impairments arising from either injury-related causes or other causes. The number includes 3566122 people with a loss, deformity or impairment of an upper extremity and 5909752 with a loss, deformity or impairment of a lower limb.

Data from Ghana indicated that 6.0 persons per 1000 were still living with a disability (i.e. an inability to perform their usual activities) from an injury that had occurred more than one year previously (*74*); the prevalences in the urban and rural areas were 6.7 and 5.0 per 1000 respectively. Only injuries caused by blunt and penetrating mechanisms were reported. If injuries caused by burns and snakebites had been included, the estimated prevalence would have been approximately 15% higher.

3.6.4 *Potential sources of further data*

More refined estimates of incidence, consistent with the definitions described above, are potentially available from several countries. In particular, uniform hospital discharge data are available for several defined geographical regions in Australia, Israel, New Zealand, North America and Europe, and for certain parts of Central and South America. It will be necessary, however, to query these databases using the uniform definition of limb traumas adopted by the working group. Data on injuries that do not result in hospitalization are less readily available but can be obtained from some countries through emergency department registration or surveillance systems. Data from special surveys are less common and are often limited in scope, providing insufficient information to permit the derivation of estimates of incidence or prevalence.

3.6.5 *Recommendations for making estimates of incidence and prevalence rates of the global burden*

The Working Group on Limb Trauma recommends that the following steps be taken to complete the development of global estimates of the incidence and prevalence of limb traumas.

First, for the eight WHO regions, a selected number of countries or regions within countries should be identified as Limb Trauma Study Areas. Working with the International Collaborating Centre on Injury Statistics (ICE), data should be obtained from these countries as outlined below and then used to derive global estimates within and across regions.

Second, for each of these countries the current inventory of databases should be expanded to include population-based data available from the following sources.

- *Hospital discharge data.* These are available for a defined population or geographical region. They should include at least one ICD-coded discharge diagnosis, age and gender, and preferably ICD e-codes or those from another coding scheme in order to identify the mechanism of injury.
- *Emergency department registration or surveillance systems.* These data should include at least one ICD-coded discharge diagnosis, age and gender, and preferably ICD e-codes or other codes for identifying the mechanism of injury.
- *Ongoing health surveys or one-time targeted surveys conducted within the past five years.* As a minimum these databases should include sufficient information on the nature of the injuries sustained to permit the identification of occurrences of limb trauma as defined above. The surveys may identify the occurrence of limb traumas from all causes, or they may target specific mechanisms.
- *Databases established to monitor the incidence of road traffic accidents.* As a minimum these databases should include sufficient information on the nature of the injuries sustained to permit the identification of occurrences of limb trauma as defined above.

The contents and scope of each database should be summarized, special attention being paid to its limitations in defining limb trauma. Databases available for an ongoing surveillance of the incidence of limb trauma should be identified, and the extent to which they can be used in producing data on specific indicators of limb trauma, as defined below, should be documented.

Requests should be made for data that are sufficient to allow definition of the number and rate (per 1000) of:

— hospitalizations (one or more nights) for limb trauma by age and gender;
— emergency department and outpatient visits for the acute treatment of limb trauma;
— episodes of injury resulting in medical attention or one or more days of restricted activity;
— the number of persons living with the loss, deformity or impairment of a limb as a result of trauma.

Where possible, data should be requested for the following categories: (a) age and gender; (b) location of injury, i.e. upper or lower limb; (c) nature of injury, i.e. fracture, crush, amputation, open wound, dislocation, burn or neurovascular; (d) mechanism. In addition, more detailed information regarding the location of fracture should be obtained. Uniform definitions should be provided so as to maximize the comparability of data obtained in different countries.

4. Severity and course of the conditions

4.1 Introduction

The conditions considered by the Bone and Joint Decade are all potentially severely incapacitating, but they present with a large variety of impairment and disability and cannot be viewed as a single entity. On the basis of expert opinion, this part of the report considers in depth the various characteristics of disease severity and proposes a useful model to describe the course of each condition. As a basis for discussion a preliminary template has been amended to fit each condition (Figure 4).

This difficult task involved distinguishing several profiles. Some conditions progress across a continuum: patients experience various degrees of severity at one time, and progression is not always linear over time. Some conditions, such as rheumatoid arthritis, show various profiles and may present with different unpredictable episodes of flare-up. Others, for example limb traumas or osteoporotic vertebral crush fractures, show different degrees of limitations after a sudden onset or event. A reverse disease progression is not excluded in the proposed model.

Members of the Scientific Group were divided into disease (or condition) work groups based upon expertise. The experts were asked to provide a framework for each condition which would help to categorize the levels of severity. This necessitated identifying the stages of severity. The experts had to rely on the best standardization available, using the most accepted classification or criteria in use at the start of

Figure 4
Model of the course of a musculoskeletal condition with and without interventions

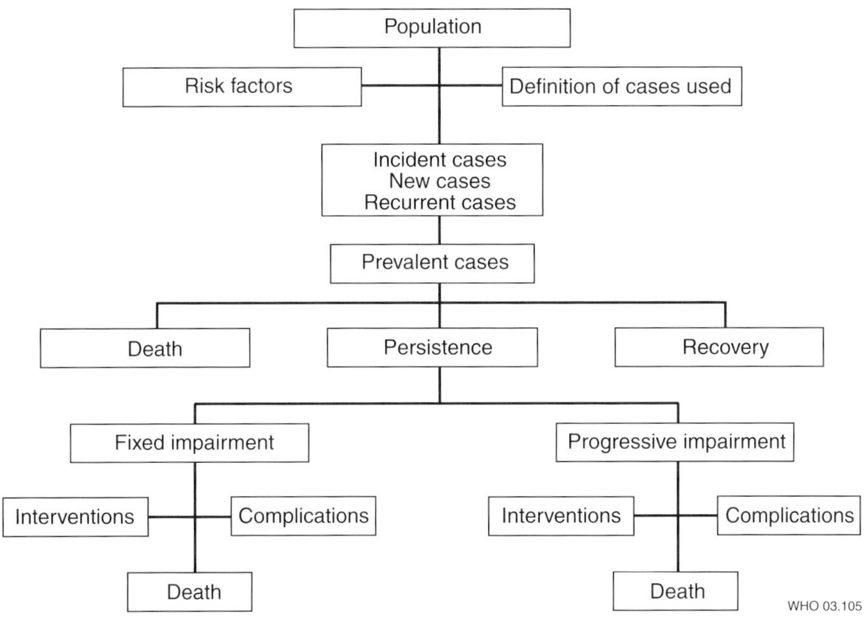

the Bone and Joint Decade. Sometimes, therefore, they had to choose between multiple existing criteria or incompletely standardized international systems. Where a standard staging was lacking, they were asked to recommend steps for creating an accessible staging system.

The task was complicated by the crucial need to make the framework available and usable where many patients do not have access to medical technology, e.g. basic X-ray or routine laboratory techniques, making it impossible to collect data in large populations during the decade. In order to ensure global applicability, the experts were advised to create aggregates or if necessary to simplify validated systems. Further difficulties arose because clinical signs and symptoms can be perceived differently in different cultures. For example, headache may be considered either a spiritual manifestation or a purely organic manifestation.

It was also intended to update the list of standardized indicators that could be used to classify health conditions and to assess the impact and consequences of the conditions. Data permitting the description of the distribution of severity are, however, scarce, since most health instruments in use have been restricted to intervention studies such as randomized controlled trials and are rarely incorporated into epidemiological studies.

In summary, the disease groups were given the following tasks:

- to reach agreement on the most suitable framework for modelling and to describe the severity of the conditions with the aim of establishing a link with prevalence and/or incidence;
- to describe the health loss in each condition, both overall and in terms of its economic impact;
- to identify possible differences in impact according to the geographical and socioeconomic environment.

It is particularly important to consider the latter point, as the perception of the conditions and their impact on patients' lives may vary greatly between societies and cultures. WHO's International Classification of Functioning and Disability (ICIDH-2) (Figure 5) offers a good opportunity to adapt the assessment of the consequences of conditions to the local individual and societal environment (restriction of participation).

In this connection the key areas for research are:

- the identification of locations where there is a need for surveys involving the use of standardized forms for the collection of data describing the distribution of severity;
- the validation of updates to the proposed classification and staging, especially if revisions are to be made during the Bone and Joint Decade;
- the routine incorporation into epidemiological studies of health instruments, most of which have been used only in intervention studies, e.g. randomized control trials;
- an invitation from GBD 2000 for expert opinion to make extrapolations from the few data available, as data on the distribution of severity are not available for most conditions;
- the modelling of the severity of juvenile rheumatoid arthritis in accordance with the recent agreement on criteria to be used for classification;
- the urgent collection of information from developing countries, as most data on health loss come from developed countries.

4.2 Rheumatoid arthritis

4.2.1 *Model of the condition*

Modelling the course of a musculoskeletal condition with or without interventions was discussed on the basis of proposing a preliminary model allowing for the reclassification of patients with persisting dis-

Figure 5
Current understanding of interactions between dimensions of ICIDH-2

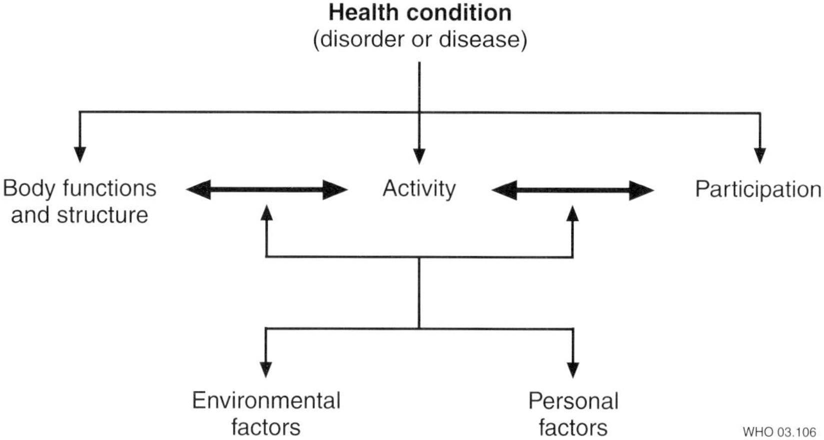

ease whose disease regresses. In addition, interventions were to be permitted at any stage of the model. There is a need for the follow-up of rheumatoid arthritis cohorts at regular intervals in order to identify the incidence of the disease and its clinical history, and it is important to assess the number of patients who move from one stage of the model to the next. Some information is available regarding (a) the incidence, prevalence and excess mortality of the disease, (b) the number of patients whose disease progresses and who recover, and (c) the types of intervention and their related complications However, such information suffers from the limitations discussed above. For ethical reasons a model of the natural history of rheumatoid arthritis that is not subject to intervention can be derived only from historical data. On the other hand, the introduction of combination therapy and the discovery of new and potent biological modifiers of inflammation may make it necessary to redefine the course of the disease. Juvenile rheumatoid arthritis cannot be considered in this model. In developing countries, a model to be used in longitudinal epidemiological studies should be designed to follow up atypical cases of arthritis which possibly evolve into classical rheumatoid arthritis (*76*).

In terms of staging and grading rheumatoid arthritis, the currently used Steinbrocker's functional capacity and radiographic assessment (*77*) has significant limitations. Steinbrocker's stages are not really useful, because the clinical data are ill-defined and some stages are too broad. The following categories could be considered for rheumatoid arthritis staging:

— the degree of inflammation (from laboratory examinations and dynamic imaging);
— structural damage (using traditional imaging techniques such as X-rays, ultrasound, magnetic resonance imaging and computerized tomography);
— clinical damage (objective findings);
— function;
— severity of clinical outlook (the speed of disease progression, extra-articular manifestations and composite indices).

At least three categories of the above components should be included in a grading system:

— functional status assessed by a self-reporting standardized questionnaire;
— anatomical damage evaluated by radiography or clinical examination (deformity);
— rate of change (pace), because the rapidity of progression of rheumatoid arthritis may vary between patients.

The staging system should be simple, inexpensive, easy to assess in the clinical setting and, ideally, applicable to epidemiological field studies. The system should combine clinical and radiographic data but should also work in a simplified form with clinical data only. This simplified version could be used where X-rays are not available. A four-step grading system (ranging from 1 = mild to 4 = severe) is probably the most appropriate form. Relevant information should be obtained by examining a limited set of joints. The hand, i.e. the proximal interphalangeal joints, the metacarpophalangeal joints and the wrist, is one of the ideal locations, although there are suggestions that rheumatoid arthritis may involve the foot at an earlier stage.

4.2.2 *How has loss of health been described and quantified?*

Both generic and disease-specific measures have been used in the assessment of health status. Most published studies have used the Health Assessment Questionnaire (HAQ) and SF-36, which have the advantage of being applicable to diseases other than rheumatoid arthritis, thus allowing a comparison of health levels in different conditions. Data exist on health resource utilization by people with rheumatoid arthritis, e.g. the number of hospitalization days, outpatient visits and invalidity pensions, but these derive mainly from industrialized countries where health expenditure is high.

4.2.3 *What is the role of geographical and socioeconomic factors?*

As discussed above, variations in the epidemiology of rheumatoid arthritis and its clinical features may occur in different areas of the world and even in the same country as a consequence of genetic and environmental factors (*78*). Not all measurements may be acceptable in each country because of differing social and cultural traditions. There are, for example, difficulties in assessing and differentiating pain in languages other than English. Fortunately, methods are available for the transcultural adaptation of health measurement instruments in different regions of the world (*79*). It was recommended that WHO endorse a battery of instruments in order to assess disease burden in musculoskeletal conditions. Finally, the point was made that patients should be involved in decisions about their disease, particularly in determining priorities in rheumatoid arthritis.

4.3 Osteoarthritis

4.3.1 *Model of the condition*

For global use we recommend a definition of osteoarthritis that is symptom-based: osteoarthritis is a condition characterized by use-related joint pain experienced on most days in any given month, for which no other cause is apparent.

The discussions were confined to peripheral joint (non-spinal) osteoarthritis.

Relatively little is known about the natural history of osteoarthritis, which varies according to the joint affected (knee, hip or hand). However, a slow progression of the radiographic evidence of joint damage and a gradual increase in the amount of pain and physical disability experienced are features generally accepted as indications of progressive osteoarthritis. Many cases do not progress, and there is also a very limited relationship between the degree of radiological change and the impact on the patient.

The radiographic stages can be defined. The following three stages are usually recognized for the purposes of identifying the burden of disease.

- *Mild*: Kellgren & Lawrence X-ray grade 0 or 1.
- *Moderate*: Kellgren & Lawrence X-ray grade 2 or 3.
- *Severe*: Kellgren & Lawrence X-ray grade 4.

Because X-rays are not available in all parts of the world, a staging system based on symptoms or physical findings would be preferable. Unfortunately, no such instrument has been validated. Options include using the ACR functional class system, which simply classifies people into five categories according to their ability to live independently with or without help, ranging from being able to do anything they want without any assistance to being so disabled that they cannot carry out simple tasks of daily living such as washing, eating or walking without major assistance. Systems such as the Joint Alignment and Motion Scale (*80*), which uses joint mobility and alignment for the clinical staging of osteoarthritis, could be adapted, but reproducibility is poor and the relationship to the impact on the patient is uncertain.

4.3.2 *How has loss of health been described and quantified?*

There are extensive data from community-based surveys in developed countries on the prevalence of joint pain, physical disability and radiographic change. All these findings are very common and strongly age-related, but the association between structural (X-ray) changes and clinical outcome is poor. There is a paucity of data from developing countries, most being reported below.

Many health instruments in use (e.g. the Western Ontario and McMaster Universities Osteoarthritis Index [WOMAC] and the Lequesne index) have been restricted to intervention studies such as randomized controlled trials. They are rarely incorporated into epidemiological studies, but the SF-36 has been used for large-scale Australian epidemiological studies (e.g. National Health Surveys). This allows comparison between disease states. Most disease reporting in these studies relies, however, on self-reporting rather than on radiographic confirmation of disease.

Data are available from developed countries on the economic consequences of work loss from osteoarthritis, on health resource utilization and on joint replacements (most of which are carried out for osteoarthritis). In Australia the total health system cost for osteoarthritis in 1993–1994 was AUS$ 624 million, which accounted for 21% of the total expenditure on musculoskeletal disease (*81*). Public and private hospitals share the greatest cost burden of osteoarthritis management (AUS$ 265 million), the cost being AUS$ 131.7 million in the public health care system and AUS$ 134.8 million in the private system. In both public and private hospitals, osteoarthritis is responsible for the greatest burden of all musculoskeletal disease on hospital expenditure (28.4% public, 28.2% private).

In Australia, osteoarthritis accounted for approximately 41 000 hospital admissions in 1993–1994, 13.9% of all hospitalizations for musculoskeletal conditions ($n = 295\,000$) (*81*). Osteoarthritis patients received the greatest number of prescriptions (3058400) in 1993–

1994, accounting for 22.9% of all prescriptions written for musculoskeletal disease (*81*). The average length of hospital stay for osteoarthritis was 9.4 days, whereas that for all musculoskeletal conditions combined was 5.0 days (*81*).

4.3.3 *What is the role of geographical and socioeconomic factors?*

Variations in the prevalence of osteoarthritis exist between countries and according to socioeconomic status, and there are also differences related to the joint site. Hip disease, for example, is less common in South-East Asian people than in Caucasians, and knee disease is more common in Blacks than in Caucasians. In developed countries, osteoarthritis is generally a greater problem among persons of comparatively low socioeconomic status than among better-off people, possibly because of an association with factors such as obesity.

4.4 Osteoporosis

4.4.1 *Model of the condition*

A classical case of osteoporosis may start in a woman about 55 years of age with a wrist fracture. Ten years later she may present with back pain, with or without minor trauma, and thoracolumbar spine X-rays may show a vertebral fracture. She might have one of several risk factors: low body weight, premature menopause, a family history of fractures, smoking, heavy alcohol consumption, inactivity, calcium or vitamin D deficiency, or corticosteroid use. The back pain may remit and relapse with subsequent vertebral fractures. Approximately 10–15 years later, at the age of 75–80 years, the patient may fall and sustain a hip fracture, resulting in hospitalization, a 20% excess risk of death, considerable functional impairment and possibly a loss of independence if she survives. Although this scenario is instantly recognizable, osteoporosis may present with any of a wide range of fractures and at a variety of ages; it is also increasingly recognized among men.

Staging and health states

WHO assigns disease burden in a similar manner for all musculoskeletal conditions; this approach commences with stages that define health states, and it provides weightings for the quality of life in each health state. Here we adapt the generic musculoskeletal model to accommodate the stages, health states and impact on the quality of life associated with the natural history of osteoporosis.

Staging

Because the risk of fracture in osteoporosis depends not only on bone fragility but also on the stochastic likelihood of trauma at different skeletal sites, it is not possible to describe stages that always evolve in a given sequence. Fractures may therefore occur in any order in a given individual. At the workshop it was decided to classify the disorder into a preclinical stage characterized by reduced bone density and a clinical stage characterized by fragility fractures. This distinction makes it possible to estimate the number of patients moving between stages and to derive risk estimates for these transitions.

Stage 1 shows a BMD T-score below –2.5 without fracture (bone loss without fracture). Stage 2 is defined by fragility fractures and postfracture health states:

- distal forearm (Colles) fracture;
- vertebral fracture;
- crush fracture syndrome;
- vertebral deformity;
- hip fracture;
- other limb fracture (e.g. proximal humeral fracture);
- fragility fractures in children.

In this classification the most common fractures are assigned a postfracture health state. A vertebral fracture in this context is one that comes to the attention of a doctor because of acute back pain leading to a spinal X-ray on which a fracture is observed. The pain and complaints relating to an acute vertebral fracture usually decrease within 6–12 months. The crush fracture syndrome, i.e. an accumulation of usually three or more vertebral fractures causing chronic pain and other complaints, is mentioned as a separate entity. When three or more vertebral fractures exist in one patient, the consequences are usually more severe and remain chronic (*82*).

Vertebral deformities form another entity and occur in patients with one or more morphometric vertebral deformities. These are recognized on X-rays, often ones obtained for other reasons. Such deformities may be asymptomatic, but quality of life studies show that the impact increases with the number of vertebral deformities (*83*). Fragility fractures in children form a special category because of the psychological and social implications and the burden on families. These fractures may occur in any order and are likely to accumulate in individuals.

The most probable order in which fractures occur is illustrated by the incidence patterns of fracture at different skeletal sites with advancing age. Thus, distal forearm or vertebral fractures typically arise first, followed by hip fractures. There are enormous geographical differences in the incidence of hip fractures, even in such a comparatively small area as Europe (see Section 3).

4.4.2 *How has loss of health been described and quantified?*

Morbidity

Health status has been described by using quality of life questionnaires. Both generic questionnaires (such as the Nottingham Health Profile [NHP], SF-36 and EuroQol EQ-5D) (*84–86*) and disease-specific questionnaires (the Quality of Life Questionnaire of the European Foundation for Osteoporosis [Qualeffo-41], Osteoporosis Assessment Questionnaire [OPAQ], Osteoporosis Quality of Life Questionnaire [OQLQ] and Osteoporosis-Targeted Quality of Life Survey Instrument [OPTQoL]) have been used for the assessment of quality of life in patients with vertebral fractures (*87–90*). Utility data can be obtained by using a preference-based questionnaire such as the EuroQol. They can be used to calculate the loss of quality-adjusted life years (QALYs). An assessment of QALYs makes it possible to compare the impacts of different diseases, e.g. osteoporosis and myocardial infarction.

Patients with a distal radius fracture have been studied longitudinally with the EuroQol questionnaire (*91*). An assessment of quality of life in patients with hip fracture is often hampered by coexisting cognitive impairment. A simple instrument for assessing quality of life in patients with hip fracture is therefore needed.

Morbidity has been assessed in a more objective way by collecting data on pain, mobility, days of bed rest and days with decreased functioning. This has been carried out in patients with vertebral fractures (*82*, *92*) and in patients with hip fractures.

Mortality

Mortality has been studied in hip fracture patients during the first year after fracture has occurred. In developed countries, mortality is high in the first year, perhaps up to 25% in women and 35% in men. Comorbidity is an important contributory factor in hip fractures and a determinant of outcome, i.e. morbidity, institutionalization in a nursing home or mortality (*93*).

4.4.3 *What is the role of geographical and socioeconomic factors?*

The impact of osteoporotic fractures on quality of life may differ between geographical regions: the prevalence of back pain in patients with vertebral fractures differs, for example, between Northern and Southern Europe and between the Netherlands and the USA. Few data are, however, available. Socioeconomic factors may also influence the impact of fractures. Whereas in the USA and Western Europe more than 90% of patients with a hip fracture are treated surgically, many patients in parts of the Russian Federation are treated by plaster cast immobilization (*94*). This has a grave impact on the quality of life, morbidity and mortality. Data on management, quality of life, morbidity and mortality related to fracture are not available for most African and Asian countries.

The following recommendations can therefore be made.

1. Health service data resources should be used to derive information on length of hospital stay, mortality, institutionalization after hip fracture and estimation of direct and indirect costs.
2. Utility data relating to both society and the patient should be obtained for hip and vertebral fractures.
3. A simple instrument for quality of life assessment in patients with hip fracture should be designed and validated.

4.5 Spinal disorders

The natural history of spinal disorders with specific causes is well described, but this is not true of nonspecific spinal disorders, which constitute more than 80% of the total. Non-comparable data have been collected for decades and are still being gathered. Consequently there is an urgent requirement for methodological standardization, the definition and inclusion of chronicity, and improved data on geographical as well as economic variables (*95–97*).

4.5.1 *Model of the conditions*

The model of the course of a musculoskeletal condition with or without interventions (Figure 4) was discussed in relation to spinal disorders. For specific spinal diseases, only slight modifications were suggested, but for nonspecific musculoskeletal spinal disorders a more novel approach is required.

A review of numerous studies suggests that the history and duration of nonspecific spinal disorders from their onset must be considered in all evaluations and studies (Table 8). It is recommended that the periods of time indicated below be used in the classification of spinal disorders.

- *Acute*: less than seven days.
- *Subacute*: more than seven days (one week).
- *Chronic*: more than 42 days (six weeks); episodes lasting more than a year should also be reported.

These categories assist in the reporting and study of nonspecific spinal disorders (*54*, *100–102*, Table 9). The use of this factor in staging also appears to demonstrate a levelling of the epidemiological data between international regions.

In addition, the uniform staging system should be simple, inexpensive and easy to assess in the clinical setting. Ideally, it should also be

Table 8
Prevalence of low back pain by age and sex

	Any LBP in past year (%)	Frequent LBP in past year (%)	Lifetime occurrence of LBP lasting more than two weeks[a] (%)
Age (years)			
18–34	61	14	10
35–49	53	21	12
50–64	56	21	18
≥65	49	18	16
Sex			
Male	53	15	14
Female	57	20	13

LBP, low back pain.
[a] The percentages are estimates because the reported age categories differed slightly from the ranges given.
Source: references *60, 98 and 99.*

applicable to epidemiological field studies. It should combine duration, symptoms, functional status, physical findings and radiographic data, but should be usable in a simplified form with clinical data alone when X-rays are not available. A four-step grading system, i.e. 1 = mild to 4 = severe, is probably the most appropriate. No validated instrument is currently available.

Specific causes
The incidence/prevalence model may, as noted above, apply to specific diseases affecting the spine, e.g. ankylosing spondylitis, radicular entrapment, scoliosis, traumatic injuries and osteoporotic crush fracture, the natural history of which is relatively uniform. A slow progression of the radiographic evidence of spinal damage and a gradual increase in the amount of pain and physical disability experienced are the generally accepted features of progressive spinal disease.

Nonspecific causes
Information on the natural history of nonspecific musculoskeletal spinal disorders is patchy. There have been no satisfactory descriptions of either the different stages of nonspecific back pain or of distinct overall course patterns (Figure 6). A simple linear model does not appear to apply to nonspecific back pain (Figure 7).

An alternative approach to staging nonspecific spinal disorders assumes a more or less unidirectional course with stable and transitional

Table 9
Classification of activity-related lumbar spinal disorders

Category	Symptoms	Duration of symptoms after onset	Working status at time of evaluation
1	Pain without radiation	a (<7 days) acute	W (working)
2	Pain + radiation to extremity, proximally	b (1–7 weeks) subacute	I (idle)
3	Pain + radiation to extremity, distally[a]	c (>7 weeks) chronic	D (disability)
4	Pain + radiation to upper/lower limb; neurological signs		
5	Presumptive compression of a spinal nerve root on a simple roentgenogram (i.e. spinal instability or fracture)		
6	Compression of spinal nerve root confirmed by specific imaging techniques (i.e. computerized axial tomography, myelography, or magnetic resonance imaging) Other diagnostic techniques (i.e. electromyography, venography)		
7	Spinal stenosis		
8	Postsurgical status 1–6 months after intervention		
9	Postsurgical status more than 6 months after intervention 9.1 Asymptomatic 9.2 Symptomatic		
10	Chronic pain syndrome		W (working)
11	Other diagnoses		I (idle)

[a] Not applicable to the cervical or thoracic segment.
Source: reproduced from reference *54* with permission of the publisher.

Figure 6
Concepts of illness

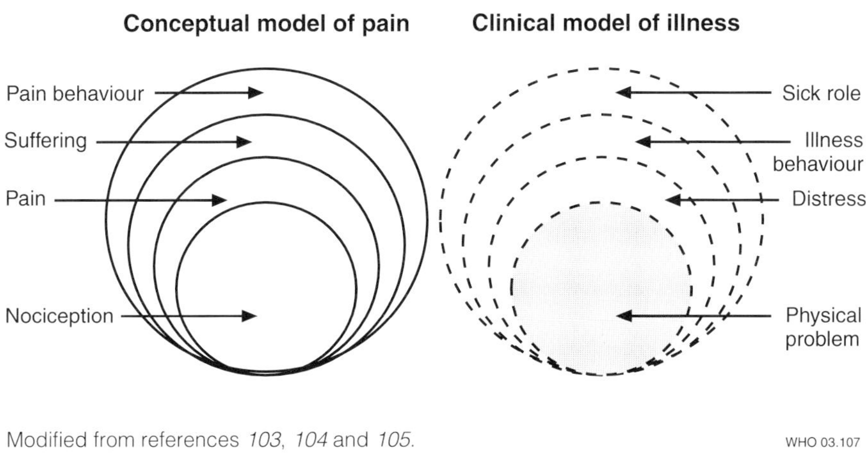

Modified from references *103*, *104* and *105*.

WHO 03.107

Figure 7
Factors affecting the pathology model of low back pain

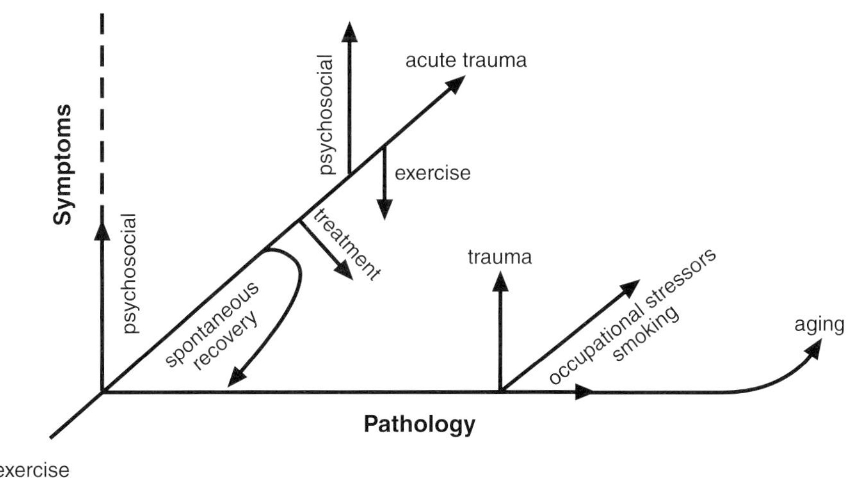

Reproduced from reference *106* with permission of the publisher.

WHO 03.108

phases from transient back pain to intermittent and finally chronic disabling back pain accompanied by increasing therapeutic requirements and a worsening overall prognosis. Such a system, similar to the tumour, node, metastases (TNM) classification for staging tumours, could support risk-adapted preventive and therapeutic strategies.

4.5.2 *How has loss of health been described and quantified?*

Both generic and disease-specific measures have been used in the assessment of health status. Many published studies have used the Sickness Impact Profile (SIP) and the SF-36 (*107*). The SF-36 is a global measure of health status and an industry standard for the assessment of health status and health outcomes. It allows a comparison of health levels across all musculoskeletal conditions.

The main descriptors of health loss caused by back pain implicitly or explicitly refer to the basic categories of ICIDH-2 (Table 10).

Health care consumption is not systematically covered by ICIDH-2 and should be assessed separately. The items to consider in this assessment are medical consultations, outpatient appointments, drugs, physiotherapy, alternative medicine and hospitalization (conservative treatment and surgical procedures), as well as simple and complex rehabilitation services.

Extensive data have been derived from community-based surveys in developed countries on the prevalence of low back pain and physical disability caused by spinal diseases and nonspecific musculoskeletal spinal disorders. All are very common and strongly age-related, but the association between structural (X-ray) changes and clinical outcome is poor. There is a paucity of data from developing countries.

In connection with the planning of a study, recall bias should be considered when data are requested for a significant time span. A recent study has suggested that individuals fail to recall episodes of low back pain within four months and may forget up to 25% of episodes of back pain for which medical care was sought because

Table 10
Health conditions resulting from musculoskeletal spinal disorders

Category	Descriptors
Impairments	Pain in the back — pain intensity, temporal characteristics and radiation/spread Concomitant problems such as other pains, somatic complaints/ somatization, distress and impaired cognition Behavioural problems
Disabilities	Activities of daily living (scale, usually assessed by questionnaire) Leisure activities Strenuous activities
Handicaps	Work disability (temporary and permanent/pension) Continually seeking help Chronic pain behaviour Dependence/care needs

of their severity (*108*). When events are forgotten, the prevalence of spinal disorders is, of course, underreported.

Not all measurements may be acceptable in all countries because of differing social and cultural traditions. There are, for example, difficulties in assessing and differentiating pain, which complicates comparison between populations. Methods are available for the transcultural adaptation of health measurement instruments and they should be adopted in different regions of the world (*70*, *71*). It was recommended that WHO endorse a battery of instruments to assess disease burden in respect of musculoskeletal conditions. Finally, the point was made that patients should be involved in decisions about their disease, particularly with regard to priorities relating to nonspecific musculoskeletal spinal disorders.

4.5.3 *What is the role of geographical and socioeconomic factors?*

The prevalence of nonspecific musculoskeletal spinal disorders varies between countries and in accordance with socioeconomic status and occupation. The more industrialized and affluent a society, the higher are the prevalences of reported back pain and back-related disability. It is not known whether this variation in prevalence and severity is a consequence of limited data collection, the limited availability of social and medical care or the identification by the cultures themselves of low back pain as a reportable medical problem. Increased reporting is most likely to be the result of cultural changes that have led to an increasing awareness of back problems, a willingness to report them and a wider acceptance of back pain as an acceptable reason for absence from work (*109*, *110*).

Recent studies (*111*, *112*) have indicated extrinsic and intrinsic risk factors for the increased incidence of nonspecific musculoskeletal spinal disorders (Table 11).

4.5.4 *Spinal pain and disability*

Further study is necessary on the chronicity of nonspecific spinal disorders because the factors leading to a chronic loss of function and, occasionally, grave disability, are not well understood. Priority should be given to investigating the loss of productivity at home or at work, the loss of quality of life and the economic impact in both the developing and industrialized countries. It seems that the factors leading to chronicity are not medical in the traditional sense but psychosocial (*53*, *113*, *114*).

The Paris Task Force (*102*) found that exercises and movements were strongly associated with improved recovery in subacute and chronic nonspecific low back pain in 13 randomized, controlled trials. Simple

Table 11
Risk factors for nonspecific musculoskeletal spinal disorders

Extrinsic Factors	Intrinsic Factors
Heavy physical labour	Anthropometrics (obesity, increased height)
Frequent bending and twisting	Spinal abnormalities
Lifting and forceful movements	Genetic predisposition
Repetitive movements	Pregnancy
Vibration	Psychosocial factors
Smoking	— psychosocial stress: self-perception
Improper body mechanics	— health beliefs: locus of control, self-efficacy, perception of disability and expectation
Insufficient exercise	— family stress
Prolonged sitting or driving	— psychological stress: somatization, anxiety and depression
	Ageing

low-cost programmes were highly successful in achieving improved function and decreased pain. Exercises and the modification of behaviour may have the strongest impact on disability. However, this is an area requiring further study. Similarly, the Quebec Task Force on whiplash-associated disorders (*115*) showed that there was no evidence in support of immobilizing the neck if no fracture or instability was present. Nonspecific musculoskeletal spinal disorders respond well to continued activity, albeit modified in the acute phase, with progressively more activation until the desired lifestyle has been achieved.

4.6 Severe limb trauma

4.6.1 *Model of the conditions*

An alternative model was proposed for limb trauma because of its acute nature (Figure 8). This framework is particularly helpful in dealing with the gamut of limb trauma incidents, regardless of treatment received or outcome. In applying it in different countries, it is important to bear in mind that patterns of care may vary substantially.

The severity of a limb trauma is generally characterized by (a) the location of the injury, (b) the type and extent of bony injury (e.g. the location and type of fracture and the extent of bone loss), and (c) the extent of soft tissue damage (i.e. muscle/tendon damage, the size of the skin defect, and neurovascular damage). Standard classifications exist for describing the nature and extent of limb traumas using these parameters. Most notable are the AO/Orthopaedic Trauma Association (OTA) classification of long bone fractures (*116*), the AO classification of soft tissue injury (*117*), the Gustilo classification of open fractures (*118*) and the Tscherne classification of closed frac-

Figure 8
Framework for limb trauma

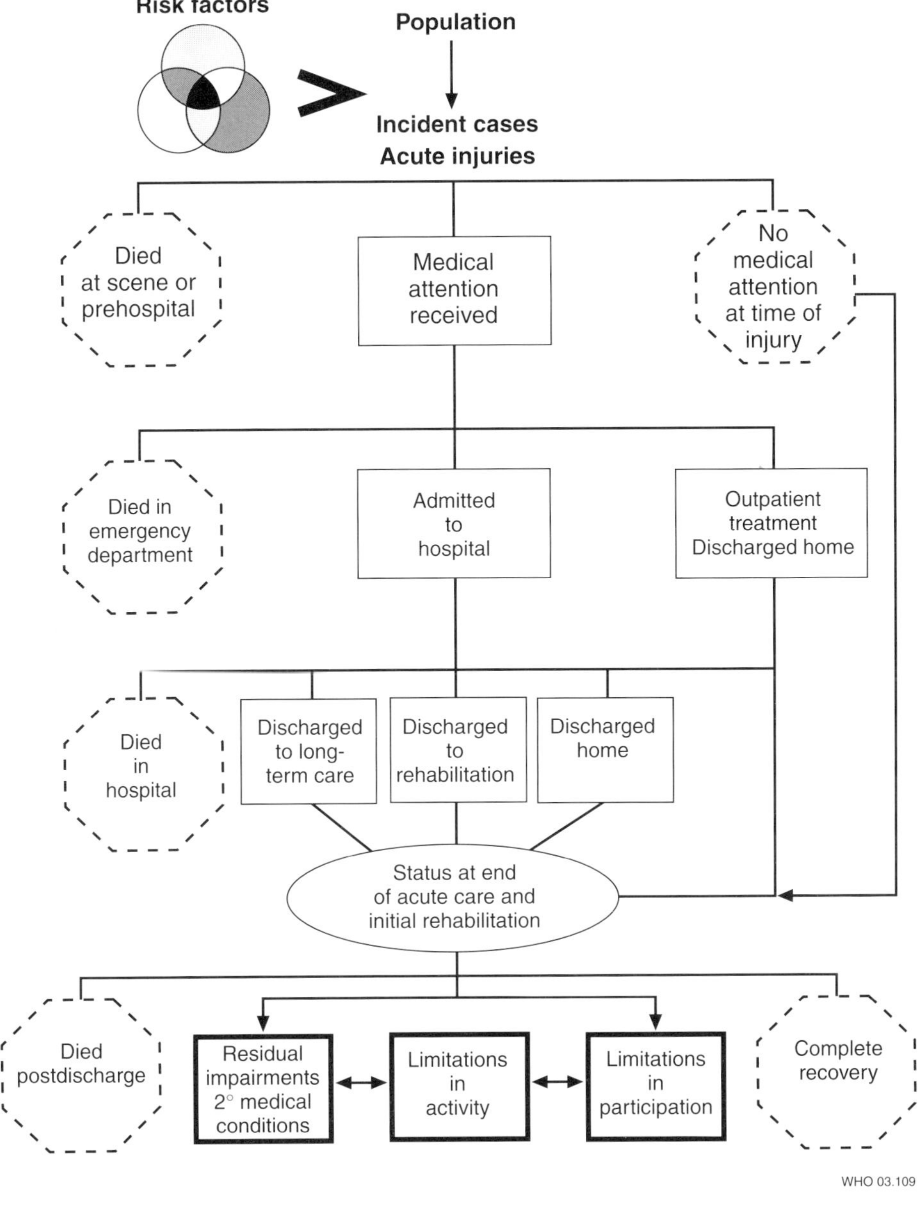

tures (*119*). These schemes are, however, relatively complex and require detailed information about the injuries which is obtained by reading X-rays.

A less complex system for rating the severity of limb injuries is provided by the Abbreviated Injury Scale (AIS) (*120*), which, although easier to use than the systems described above, is a gross measure of the severity of injuries to the extremities. On the other hand, the AIS severity can be estimated from ICD discharge diagnoses, which are routinely available in many countries (*121*). Data from the USA and other developing countries indicate that 53% of persons hospitalized for an extremity injury fall into the mild to moderate category (AIS 1–2) and that 47% fall into the severe category (AIS 3–4).

The working group made the recommendations indicated below on the classification of limb injuries and their severity.

First, consideration should be given to promoting the classification of fractures in accordance with the following scheme, which combines the Tscherne and Gustilo classifications.

- *Type A fractures* (least severe): closed Tscherne classes 0 and I.
- *Type B fractures*: open Gustilo classes I and II.
- *Type C fractures*: closed Tscherne classes II and III.
- *Type D fractures* (most severe): open Gustilo class III.

Second, the AIS should be promoted as a universal system for rating the severity of injuries, including limb injuries. Given the widespread use of ICD, AIS scores generated from ICD rubrics will be particularly useful in summarizing the incidence of limb traumas by severity across various countries that maintain administrative databases, as described above. It is necessary to develop a score based on the AIS which summarizes the effect of multiple injuries on the same extremity. As yet there are only scores covering multiple injuries across all body systems (*122*). Work is also in progress under the auspices of OTA and the American Association for the Advancement of Automotive Medicine, which developed the AIS, on revising the current AIS in order to make it more compatible with AO/OTA classifications.

Additional research is needed in order to validate existing classification systems with regard to their correlation with impairment and functional outcome. Revisions to these classifications should be made in the light of the results.

4.6.2 *How has loss of health been described and quantified?*

Although numerous reports have documented the range of short-term complications and impairments following limb trauma, few studies have examined the extent to which these impairments translate into long-term functional limitations and disability, including the inability to resume major activities such as working, going to school and maintaining a household. However, several studies have looked at the consequences of hip fractures among the elderly, with reference to functional outcome, quality of life and overall cost. Selected studies on the impact of other extremity injuries were presented to the group so as to provide some background for the monitoring project.

One study from the USA, for example, used SIP to examine the outcome for persons aged 16–69 with unilateral lower extremity trauma (*123*, *124*). Thirty months after injury, 64% had no disability (SIP score 0–3), whereas 17%, 12% and 7% had mild, moderate and severe disability respectively (SIP scores 4–9, 10–19, and 20 and above). Disability was distributed across the spectrum of activities of daily living, including physical functioning, psychosocial functioning, sleep and work. Six months after injury, 49% of those who had been working before injury had returned to work; at 12 and 30 months the corresponding values were 72% and 82%. Similar results were obtained in a cohort of patients admitted to a hospital in Denmark (*125*).

Another study in the USA indicated that significant impairment persisted seven months after injury in approximately half of persons hospitalized for a major hand injury (*126*). These impairments generally translated into poor hand functioning, and one-fifth of the patients reported significant disability. Of those who had been working before injury, 37% had not returned to work seven months after the event.

As indicated above, another study examined the impact of injuries in two populations in Ghana, in which the majority of those injured had injuries involving one or more limbs (*127*). Data were obtained on 21 100 persons. Of the 1609 injuries reported for the previous year, 13 led to fatalities (0.8% of reported injuries), 445 were severe injuries (defined as leading to a disability period of 30 days or more; 27.7% of reported injuries), and 1151 were minor injuries (a disability period of 1–29 days; 71.5% of reported injuries).

Very few studies have been published in which the outcomes of limb trauma in children are described. One study, however, indicated that injuries to the extremities accounted for one-quarter of the disabilities recorded six months after severe, multisystem injuries sustained by children aged 1–17 years (*128*).

Comprehensive studies of the economic impact of limb trauma are equally sparse. Data from the USA indicated that total medical expenditure was about US$ 11261 and US$19 748 (1985 values) per person hospitalized with upper and lower limb traumas respectively (*129*, *130*). The medical expenditure for persons treated as outpatients was considerably lower but not inconsequential (US$ 298 and

US$ 271 for upper and lower limb traumas respectively). The average comprehensive costs were estimated to be US$ 211964 and US$ 349517 for persons hospitalized with upper limb and lower limb traumas respectively. The corresponding figures for non-hospitalized patients were US$ 4261 and US$ 5382. These costs include both monetary costs (costs related to direct health care expenditures and the value of lost productivity) and an estimate of fair compensation for pain, suffering and lost quality of life. When combined with suggested figures for the annual incidence of limb traumas in the USA, estimates of the total comprehensive costs exceed US$ 144 billion for upper extremities and US$ 325 for lower extremities.

In Ghana the mean treatment cost per injury, i.e. the out-of-pocket payment for any form of treatment, supplies and drugs, for injured persons living in urban and rural environments was estimated to be US$ 31 and US$ 11 respectively for all injuries sustained during the previous year (*127*). As indicated above, however, the majority of the injuries affected the extremities (*74*). Moreover, the costs must be viewed in relation to the local minimum wage of US$ 1 per day. This study emphasizes that traditional cost measures may not adequately capture the full impact of injuries in developing countries. Other measures that should be examined include labour reallocation (as over 80% of relatives took time off from their usual duties to care for injured persons), the need to borrow money (20% of injured persons borrowed money and 10% were still in debt on average four months after injury), the need to sell belongings (4% did so), reduced food production (one-third of rural families indicated that farm production had decreased) and reduced food consumption (one-quarter of families indicated that food consumption had declined).

4.6.3 *Role of geographical and socioeconomic factors*

The consequences of injury vary greatly, not only because of its nature and severity, but also in relation to whether multiple injuries to the ipsilateral or contralateral extremity are sustained, the presence and severity of injuries to other body systems, the age of the injured person, the presence of pre-existing chronic conditions and health-related habits such as smoking and alcohol use, and other non-medical risk factors related to the person and the physical, work, social and economic environment. In some cultures the extent to which disability compensation is received can also be an important predictor of return to work and overall recovery.

The relative importance of these factors in relation to outcome has not been well characterized because most studies focus on only one factor at a time and because of a failure to incorporate objective measures of physical impairment into analyses. Only a few studies have examined the non-medical factors influencing outcome after limb injury (*127*, *131–133*). Less information is available on geographical differences in the consequences of limb injuries. However, wide variations can be expected, related to differences in access to immediate acute care, rehabilitation, prosthetic devices and adaptive equipment.

5. Health and economic indicators

5.1 The need for health indicators

The issue of bone and joint problems highlights the need for health indicators that capture the entire profile of people with health conditions involving these states. It is increasingly recognized that one needs to look beyond the traditional parameters of diagnosis and mortality and to examine measures of functioning and disability as well as the quality of life. This makes it possible not only to understand the health states in their entirety but also to address the positive aspects of health. It is necessary to create a common language and a common metric for functioning and disability that will enable us to communicate better when talking about health outcomes that are non-fatal or health states that are less than perfect.

A summary measure of health combines information on both mortality and morbidity by means of a parsimonious set of domains. Imagine, for example, that a person develops a health condition at the age of 30 years and that this leads to an overall decline in health to 40% of the original state of perfect health (as measured via this parsimonious set of health domains). Subsequently, some interventions are made and adaptations occur, resulting in partial improvement until a terminal illness leads to death. In this situation the summary measure is the area under the life curve.

It is necessary to consider how to calculate this and how to aggregate the measures from individuals to the level of the population. Information is needed on the nature of the disease in question, obtainable from the ICD, currently in its tenth revision, and on functioning and disability, obtainable from the International Classification of Functioning, Disability and Health (ICF), which represents a revision of the previously abbreviated classification scheme ICIDH that was first published in 1980.

ICD focuses mainly on diagnosis. It provides the framework for reporting diseases, disorders or injuries and underlying conditions, as well as for documenting their processes and etiologies. ICF captures information on functioning and disability and provides the framework for describing how a person's body functions, what he or she can do in usual daily activities, ranging from simple to complex, and what his or her actual participation or involvement is in these areas, in relation to the prevailing environment.

Diagnosis alone fails to predict health care needs, but the addition of information on functioning and disability makes it possible to achieve better prediction of health service utilization, the length of hospitalization, the improvement in functioning after hospitalization, return to work, work performance and the recovery of social integration. ICF can therefore provide a very useful framework for health care policy and decision-making on the identification of needs, the targeting of interventions, the measurement of outcomes, the effectiveness of interventions, the setting of priorities and the allocation of resources.

By using a common language, ICF can also serve as a link with related sectors such as those of education and welfare. It provides a scientific basis for the description of non-fatal health outcomes and for documenting the consequences of health conditions. The common language allows comparison between countries of health states that are less than perfect, and between health care disciplines, services and different periods. It provides a systematic coding scheme that can be used in health information systems for automated processing.

ICF views functioning and disability as occurring at several different levels. First, it is possible to consider the impairments that can occur in the functions and structures of the body as a significant deviation or loss. At the second level, ICF views functioning in terms of the individual's activities and the limitations on them. This can also be understood as the capacity of the individual to carry out a task or action in a standard or uniform environment, whereby an assessment of ability can be made which takes account of the environment and thus reflects the person's health status. At the third level, ICF views the person's functioning in society, i.e. his or her participation, formerly viewed in terms of handicap. This means considering whether the person is involved in community activities. A problem in participation is called a restriction. This can also be understood as the real-life performance of the individual, i.e. what the individual does in the actual environment in which he or she lives, with all its facilitators and barriers.

A person in a wheelchair may, for example, have an impairment of decreased power in both lower limbs (body function level) that has resulted from a spinal cord injury. Such a person has a decreased capacity to move and is thus limited in the activity of moving from place to place (person-level functioning). If there are no ramps in the buildings in the person's environment, he or she experiences heightened difficulty in moving around. Consequently, real-life performance is worse than the capacity possessed by the person (society-level functioning), a clear restriction on participation imposed by the environment. A clinician or a rehabilitation therapist may be concerned with the impairment or capacity/activity limitations, whereas consumer organizations and activists may be concerned with problems of participation. The classification thus provides a common language that allows translation between different user groups. It also allows identification of what can be done for individuals and their environment so as to enhance functioning. Furthermore, it allows the effects of these interventions to be measured.

The ICF model is interactive, and a health condition may result in an impairment of body function or structure, limitations of activity or restrictions of participation that are independent of each other. This model also considers personal and environmental contextual factors. ICF has undergone extensive field tests. Assessment tools have been developed for users at different levels, ranging from patient assessments and population surveys to reporting from clinical information systems.

A major shift in thinking on functioning and disability reflected in ICF lies in its universal and etiologically neutral approach. It is applied to all people and does not assume any causal relationships. It thus brings parity across health conditions since it uses functioning and disability as the common metric for assessing the impact of health conditions and looks at the effects on the individual rather than at the causes.

ICF can form the framework for outcome measurement and can evaluate the difference that can be made to people's lives during the Bone and Joint Decade. Outcomes are multidimensional. The choice of indicators depends on the purpose for which they are being used. It may vary in accordance with whether they arise from the perspective of the person with the health condition, the caregivers, the providers or the state. The outcome measures may be signs and symptoms of disease or indicators of functioning and disability. Furthermore, it may be desired to consider the subjective appraisal of the health state, i.e. the quality of life or subjective well-being associated with the condition in question as an additional measure of the overall health experience.

WHO's Disability Assessment Schedule (WHODAS II, originally WHO-DAS) has been developed as a measure that is linked to the conceptual framework of ICF. It has undergone extensive qualitative and quantitative testing on samples of clinical and general populations in different cultural settings. It has six domains: understanding and communication, getting around, self-care, getting along with people, life activities and participation in society. The scoring system includes ratings of the difficulties of carrying out several different tasks or actions as well as of the number of days in the past month when the difficulties have been present. There is a fully structured version for epidemiological surveys, a clinical semistructured version for use in clinical encounters, and proxy versions for use by clinicians or family members.

The ICF framework, in conjunction with the linked measurement tools, will provide a robust set of tools for the measurement of disability and less-than-perfect health states contributing to the burden of different health conditions. In this manner, diseases do not have to be viewed as being single homogeneous entities but can be realistically categorized as mild, moderate or severe. Furthermore, disability can also be evaluated in relation to the two separate dimensions of intensity and duration. Minimum data sets can be identified from the ICF categories for use in connection with a variety of health conditions and health settings.

When decisions involving resource allocation (or those which have other economic implications) are being made, it is important to understand the value that people attach to different health states. These values can be measured by determining people's preferences or choices with the help of various techniques, e.g. those of willingness to pay, standard gamble, time trade-off and person trade-off. A combination of the descriptive and valuation measurements can be used to assign disability weights to health states, which can then be used to compute summary measures of health such as DALYs. These summary measures can be used for comparing the cost-effectiveness of different interventions for a range of health conditions, and this analysis can assist policy-makers in setting priorities.

In summary, ICF aims to provide a scientific basis for classifying the consequences of various health conditions and serves as a common language bridging the medical and social models of disability. Importantly, it places health in the context of human development by focusing on functionality, productivity and social participation. It is intended to be practical and easy to use, as well as relevant and useful in measuring differences in health.

5.2 What should be measured by indicators for musculoskeletal conditions?

The word "indicator" signifies a broad range of parameters that measure the impact of musculoskeletal diseases on individuals, populations and society. The need for health indicators for musculoskeletal conditions has already been emphasized, with reference to the operationalization of health indicators by means of ICF. The indicators should include not only basic demographic parameters but also measures of the quality of life, the availability and provision of specific treatments for musculoskeletal conditions, and the environmental factors and risk factors influencing the onset and outcomes of these conditions.

There is a wide range of indicators and many more instruments that can be used to measure the various domains. The indicators may be categorized as:

- general indicators, including demographic parameters;
- risk factors, including environmental factors;
- specific interventions and treatments;
- consequences of musculoskeletal conditions for the individual and society.

5.2.1 *General indicators*

Demographic data such as those on age and sex are important as indicators of musculoskeletal conditions. The variation in age bands used in different studies and reports sometimes makes it difficult to pool information or to make comparisons between countries. The age bands used by WHO should be evaluated for their suitability in relation to musculoskeletal disorders.

Indicators on culture and ethnicity are important in terms of both possible risk factors and the potential consequences of musculoskeletal conditions for the individual. The inability to cycle or squat, for example, has very different consequences for individuals in different parts of the world. The instruments to be used may vary between regions, countries or continents. It is evident that the instruments employed can provide only a rough indication of cultural and ethnic factors, as can those that measure socioeconomic status. The latter indicator is important as it plays a role both as a risk factor for musculoskeletal conditions and in affecting their outcome. This is also true for comorbidity, which is very hard to record with a single measure.

5.2.2 *Risk factors*

Many general indicators, such as age, geographical area and socioeconomic status are also important as risk factors for musculoskeletal conditions. Additional risk factors include occupation, family history, BMI, alcohol, smoking, diet and education, and this list is still incomplete. In the case of trauma, local regulations play a role.

5.2.3 *Specific interventions and treatments*

An indication of the availability of specific interventions and treatments for musculoskeletal conditions provides an insight into what is being done and what can be done in particular situations. Many effective preventive and therapeutic interventions are available for decreasing the prevalence of severe musculoskeletal disorders. Specific interventions include health education, the introduction of regulations (e.g. on traffic and work situations), symptomatic and disease-modifying pharmacotherapeutic interventions, surgical interventions, paramedical treatments and rehabilitation. These may be measured by the availability and cost of medical visits, hospital admissions, and so on. The side-effects of therapeutic interventions should not be omitted.

5.2.4 *Consequences of musculoskeletal conditions for the individual and society*

In general, people do not die from musculoskeletal conditions. However, a decreased life expectancy is associated with some musculoskeletal disorders and with musculoskeletal conditions in people who have inadequate access to treatment and live in poor socioeconomic circumstances. Mortality from musculoskeletal disorders is hard to estimate because they have hardly been mentioned as a cause of death on death certificates.

The major impact of musculoskeletal conditions is on the quality of life. This is determined not only by illness but also by socioeconomic, personal, environmental and other factors. When discussing indicators for these disorders we need information on the quality of life in relation to illness. This can be defined as the overall impact of illness and its treatment on patients, together with their responses. The specific consequences of musculoskeletal conditions are pain, stiffness, loss of mobility of the joints, deformity, disability, loss of independence, reduced numbers of social interactions, a decline in well-being and, to a lesser degree, mortality. In line with the ICF system, the indicators can be divided into those for: (a) loss of body function and structure, (b) limitation of function and (c) restriction imposed by society.

With regard to the first category there are many instruments that can measure disease-specific loss of function and structure in musculoskeletal conditions. They measure symptoms, disease activity, joint mobility, deformity, joint damage or anatomical disease stages. The instruments include the single and composite scores for symptoms and disease activity such as the ACR, the EULAR and the DAS scores; range of motion scores, body height and flexion index that measure deformity; and radiographic scores that measure joint damage.

Limitation of function may imply restriction of the essential activities of daily living, such as standing, walking and gripping, complex activities such as self-care, discretional activities that often include strenuous exertion and activities requiring endurance, such as hobbies and sport. Essential activities can be assessed by actual measurement (walking time or grip strength) or the use of self-administered questionnaires. Complex activities of daily living are assessed by the latter means. The few good instruments available for measuring the discretional categories are mainly questionnaires.

The instruments available for measuring the activities of daily living and well-being often measure both to a varying degree. Sometimes they also measure restriction. These instruments are either developed specifically for one or more musculoskeletal conditions (disease-specific instruments) or are generic and meant to allow comparison between other chronic diseases. The capacities of instruments specifically intended for measuring musculoskeletal conditions should include measurement of the function of the upper and lower extremities, dexterity, bodily contact and body image.

Some examples of generic instruments are the SF-36 and SF-12, the Barthel Index, the SIP, the NHP, the WHODAS II and the EuroQol. Frequently used instruments that are specific for musculoskeletal conditions are the Steinbrocker classification, the HAQ, the Arthritis Impact Measurement Scales (AIMS), the Rheumatoid Arthritis-Specific Quality of Life Instrument, the ACR classification, the Keitel Function Test and the WOMAC.

Finally, restriction by society can partly be measured by some of the above-mentioned questionnaires, such as AIMS, but instruments measuring social interactions and independence are generally scarce.

5.2.5 *Choice of indicators*

A major task for the near future is to choose the most appropriate indicators for assessing the impact of musculoskeletal conditions worldwide. Among the multitude of instruments used for the assessment of such disorders in various settings, those that are simple, available, widely used, informative and appropriate to musculoskeletal conditions should be selected.

5.3 Economic indicators

Studies on the cost of illness have gained prominence in health policy circles because of their ability to compare in common terms, i.e. money, the impacts of conditions of varying prevalence and effect, including conditions such as lung cancer, which is primarily fatal, and those such as osteoarthritis, which is primarily disabling. In addition, the principal method of enumerating the cost of illness, the human capital approach, provides a way of assessing the direct impact of conditions as expenditure on medical care and the indirect effect as lost wages.

Evidence is reviewed here on the cost of musculoskeletal conditions in general and on that of rheumatoid arthritis, one of the more severe musculoskeletal disorders. Interestingly, studies on the cost of the broad gamut of musculoskeletal conditions as a whole have been derived from random samples of community-based populations and self-reporting, whereas studies on the cost of rheumatoid arthritis have been based solely on clinical samples and have involved diagnosis of this discrete condition by physicians.

The most recent comprehensive study of the cost of musculoskeletal conditions related to 1995 (*134*). Overall, the direct cost amounted to US$ 88.7 billion, of which the largest component, US$ 33.7 billion or 38%, was attributable to hospital admissions (Figure 9). Nursing home admissions accounted for the next largest component (21%), and physicians' visits accounted for 17% of the total. In the USA, administrative costs are another relatively large component, viz. US$ 4.7 billion or about 5% of the total. The indirect cost was far larger, amounting to US$ 126.2 billion (Figure 10), or 58% of the total cost of US$ 214.9 billion. Since musculoskeletal conditions are rarely fatal, only 7% of the 58% of the total cost attributable to wage losses arose from premature mortality, the remaining 51% resulting from morbidity.

The 1995 study (*123*) was the latest in a series that the author and her colleagues had conducted into the cost of musculoskeletal conditions.

Figure 9
Direct cost of musculoskeletal conditions in the USA, by type, 1995

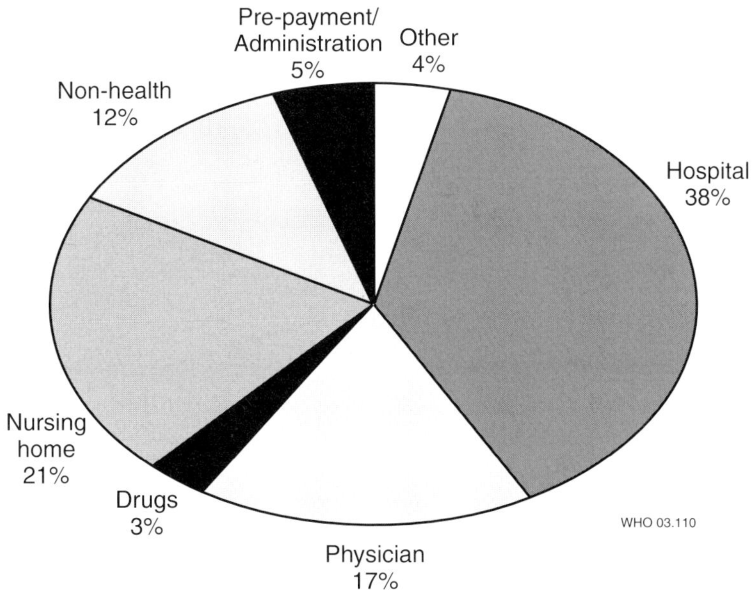

Total direct costs were US$ 88.7 billion. "Non-health" includes transportation, household help, alterations to the home, etc.

Source: reference *135*.

Figure 11 shows the time trend in these studies, expressed as the percentage of gross domestic product (GDP) for each year. In 1963 the total cost of musculoskeletal conditions was about 0.5% of GDP, split approximately equally between direct medical care costs and indirect wage loss costs. In 1972 the overall cost had grown slightly as a percentage of GDP; a much larger growth had occurred in the wage loss portion because of rising real incomes. The total cost did not grow much between 1972 and 1980, but because this was a period of wage stagnation and rapid medical care inflation, there was a much faster increase in the proportional cost of medical care. In subsequent years the cost rose precipitously: the total outlay associated with musculoskeletal conditions reached 2.5% of GDP in 1992 and almost 3% in 1995. Musculoskeletal conditions thus had the same economic impact as a severe and chronic economic slow-down, as the economy is said to be in recession when it contracts by 1% for three consecutive quarters.

Figure 12 shows the direct and indirect costs associated with musculoskeletal conditions by age in 1995. Since persons aged 18 years and

Figure 10
Total cost of musculoskeletal conditions in the USA, 1995

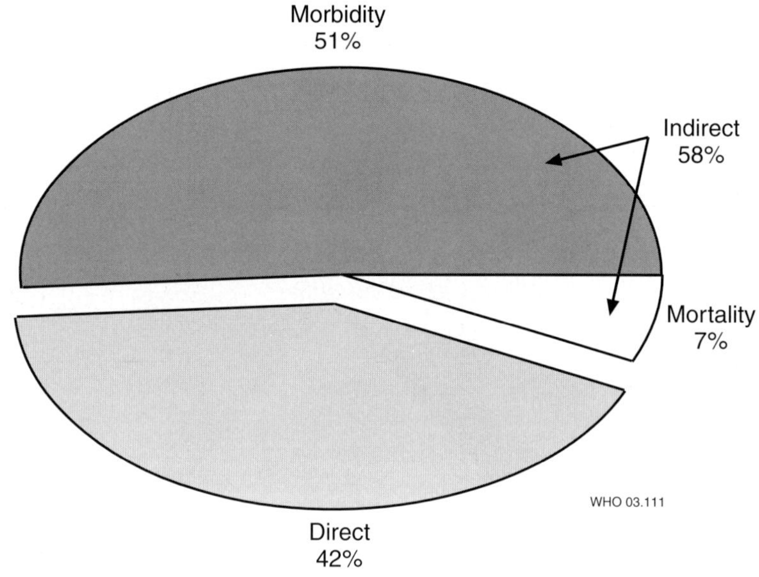

Total costs were US$ 214.9 billion.

Reproduced from reference *135* with permission of the publisher.

Figure 11
Direct and indirect cost of musculoskeletal conditions as a percentage of gross domestic product, by year

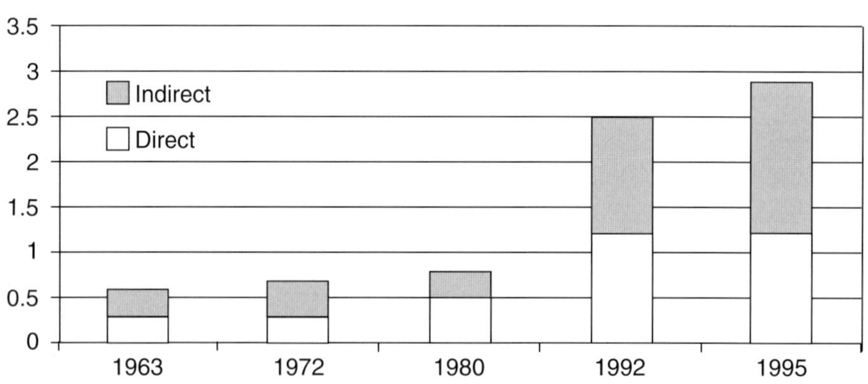

Source: reference *136*.

WHO 03.112

Figure 12
Direct and indirect cost of musculoskeletal conditions, in US$ billions, by age, 1995

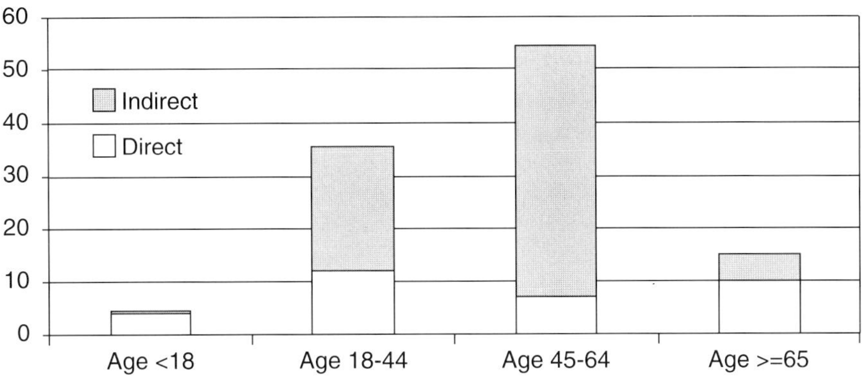

Source: reference *135*.

WHO 03.113

younger are not expected to work, almost all their cost is associated with medical care expenditure, as is most of the cost for persons aged 65 years and over. On the other hand, most of the cost for persons aged 18–44 and 45–64 years arises from lost income. Interestingly, the total cost for persons aged less than 65 years is much smaller than that of the older age group, belying the notion that the economic impact is concentrated on older people.

Of the total cost of US$ 214.9 billion for musculoskeletal conditions in 1995, a cost of US$ 82.4 billion was associated with arthritis, the most prevalent forms of which were osteoarthritis and rheumatoid arthritis (Figure 13). Of the total cost for arthritis, the direct cost amounted to US$ 21.7 billion, or about 26%, the remaining US$ 60.8 billion arising from lost wages. Of the total cost, nursing homes accounted for 15% (59% of the direct cost), and hospital care accounted for 4% (14% of the direct cost).

The sizeable literature on the economic impact of rheumatoid arthritis has been reviewed (*137*). The studies show that at least 75% of the total cost of this illness arises indirectly from the relatively high rate of work disability. Moreover, the range of costs is remarkably similar: the direct costs range from US$ 4000 to US$ 6000 per year in constant dollars, and the indirect costs range from US$ 12000 to US$ 24000. Of the direct costs, between 40% and 60% are attributable to hospital admissions, even though only about 10% of persons with rheumatoid arthritis are hospitalized for the condition in any year. Overall, therefore, the two most expensive items in the costs of rheumatoid arthritis are wage losses and hospital care.

Although large, the direct cost of rheumatoid arthritis is highly skewed (Table 12). The median total direct cost is only about US$ 2715 per year. The median cost for physician visits is only US$ 416, whereas the median drug cost is US$ 1206. However, the total direct cost can be as high as US$ 85469 a year, the hospital cost alone accounting for as much as US$ 81998. Indeed, although drugs

Figure 13
Direct and indirect cost of arthritis in the USA, 1995

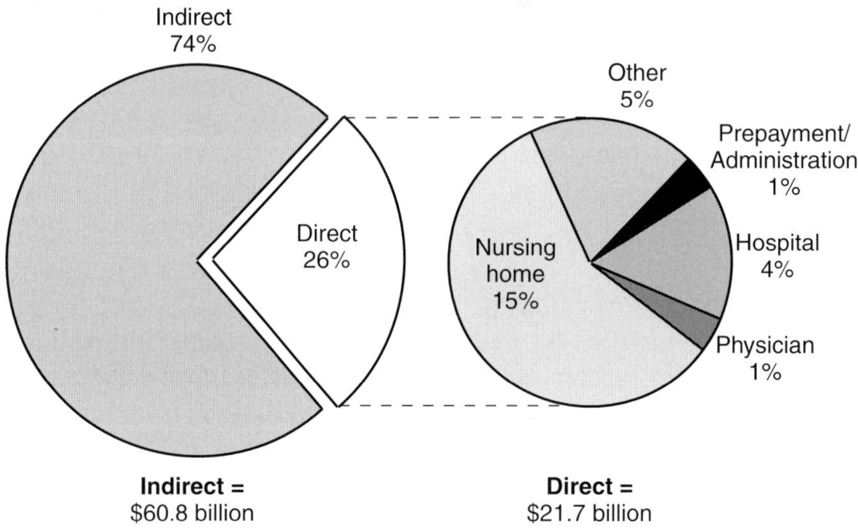

Total costs were US$ 82.4 billion.

WHO 03.114

Source: reference *136*.

Table 12
Highly skewed direct cost of rheumatoid arthritis

Type of cost	Mean (US$)	Median (US$)	Maximum (US$)
Hospital	3061	0	81998
TJR admissions	1533	0	51926
Other surgical admissions	1098	0	67617
Medical admissions	149	0	29694
Physician visits	511	416	13528
Drugs	1552	1206	5409
Total	**5919**	**2715**	**85469**

TJR, total joint replacement.
Reproduced from reference *137* with permission of the publisher.

Figure 14
Distribution of health costs, by type, in high-cost and low-cost patients

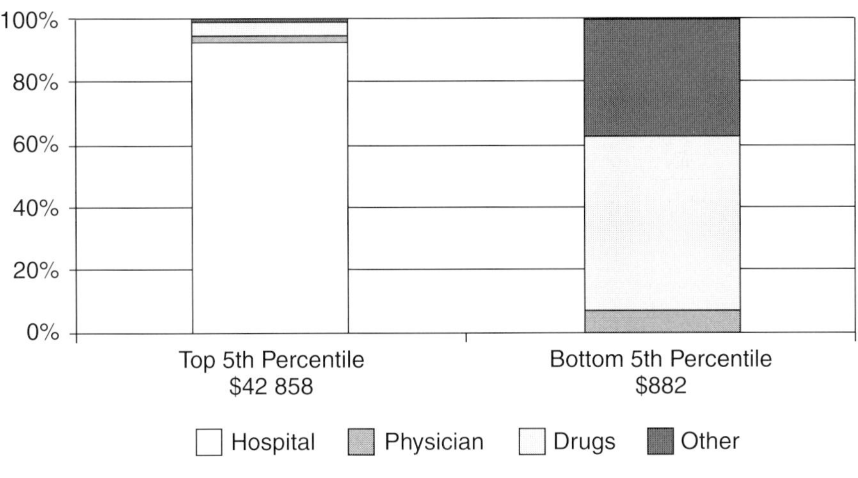

Hospital costs are dominant in the highest quintile, while drug costs are highest in the lowest quintile.

Source: reference *136*.

WHO 03.115

Table 13
Comparison of skewness of ten-year to one-year direct cost of rheumatoid arthritis

	Mean (US$)	Median (US$)	Maximum (US$)	Ratio of Median/Maximum
One-Year	5919	2715	85469	3%
Ten-Year	57201	41113	191540	22%

Adapted from reference *137* with permission of the publisher.

dominate the cost profile of persons in the bottom fifth percentile of expenditure (Figure 14), the hospital cost dominates the profile of those in the top 20%, again suggesting that in order to save a significant amount of money, it would be prudent to reduce the hospital admission rate.

Although the cost in any one year is highly skewed, the long-term cost is much less so (Table 13). Thus, in any year the median cost of US$ 2715 is about 3% of the maximum cost of US$ 85469, whereas over a 10-year period the median cost of US$ 41113 is 22% of the maximum cost of US$ 191540. In the long term, therefore, individuals are increasingly likely to experience a high cost.

Figure 15
Summarising scenarios of the impact of gender on the per person indirect cost of rheumatoid arthritis

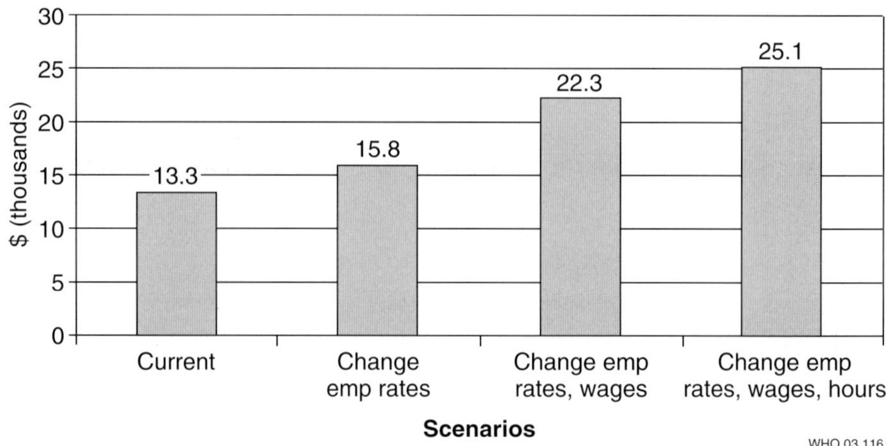

Because the indirect cost plays such an important role in determining the total cost of musculoskeletal conditions in general and rheumatoid arthritis in particular, it is important to understand how the contemporary labour markets affect estimates of the wage loss associated with these conditions. Studies of the indirect cost of illness are based on the assumption that, in the labour market, wages are determined fairly, i.e. they are not subject to discrimination on the basis of gender, race or health status. If, however, a racial minority is relegated to low-paying jobs relative to their training and experience, the estimated cost of wage losses attributable to illnesses with a higher prevalence in the group will be relatively low. Potentially, this deprives the condition in question of a fair allocation for treatment and research. Because musculoskeletal conditions occur disproportionately among women, a gender discrimination in employment may lead to underestimation of the economic impact of the conditions. In fact, women have a lower employment rate than men, and when they are employed they work fewer hours and receive less pay than men.

Figure 15 summarizes three scenarios of the impact of gender on the indirect cost of rheumatoid arthritis per person. In the first, women and men have an equal employment rate; in the second, they have an equal employment rate and equal wages and in the third, they have an equal employment rate, equal wages and equal hours. Compared with the proposal that the indirect cost averages US$ 13300 without correction for bias, these scenarios result in an increase in indirect cost of

US$ 15 800, US$ 22 300 and US$ 25 100 respectively. Thus, the estimate of indirect cost for the third scenario, which takes employment rate, hours and earnings into account, may be almost twice the initial estimate of US$ 13 300.

5.4 Summary

The cost of musculoskeletal conditions would appear to be growing with the ageing of the population and the increased utilization of new medical technologies. It is now approaching 3% of GDP. This is equivalent to a permanent severe recession. The economic impact of rheumatoid arthritis, a common severe form of arthritis, is in the range of US$ 4000–6000 per case for direct cost and US$ 12 000–24 000 for indirect cost. Large though this indirect cost is, it may be an underestimate because of gender bias in the labour market.

6. Measuring the health impact and economic burden of musculoskeletal conditions on the population

6.1 Introduction

As indicated in earlier sections, the burden of musculoskeletal conditions can be measured by counting how many people exhibit them. However, this does not reveal how the conditions affect individuals, their ability to function, their families and society in general.

There is a need to identify indicators for the measurement of risk of disease or injury and of health impact which are applicable to all the musculoskeletal conditions being studied. This section considers indicators that could be used for assessing the impact of musculoskeletal conditions on populations, collected either as routine health statistics or in surveys. Section 7 considers domains and indicators that describe the health status of the individual which can also be used to monitor populations.

A range of possible indicators has been considered for application to the various populations of the world. Their relevance to the different musculoskeletal conditions being reviewed has been assessed (Table 14). The current or potential availability of such indicators has also been considered for different geographical populations. These indicators are tabulated so as to show whether the data are already available or whether it would be feasible to collect them in developed or developing countries (Tables 15 and 16). Such indicators could be

Table 14

Indicators of risk and impact relevant to different musculoskeletal conditions[a]

Indicator relevant for:	Conditions					
	Rheumatoid arthritis	Osteo-arthritis	Osteoporosis	Osteoporosis with fracture	Back pain and other spinal disorders	Major limb trauma
Risk factors						
Smoking	±	±	+	+	+	–
Alcohol	±	±	+	+	–	+
Body mass index	+	+	+	+	+ and –	–
Family history	±	+	+	+	+	–
Corticosteroid use			+	+		
Thyrotoxicosis			+	+		
Previous fracture			+	+		
Immobility			+	+	+ and –	
Heavy physical or repetitive activity					±	
Impact						
Independence/disability						
Activities of daily living/essential self-care	+	+	–	+	+	+
Complex activities of daily living/leisure activities	±	±	–	±	+	+
Quality of life						
Physical dimension	+	+	–	+	+	+
Mental dimension/psychological well-being	+	±	–	±	+	+
Social dimension	+	±	–	+	+	+

Work loss						
Disability pension	+	+	−	+	+	+
Worker compensation	+	+	−	+	+	+
Mortality						
Related to condition or intervention	+	−	±	+	±	+
Resource utilization						
Number of visits						
Physician	+	+	±	+	+	+
Consultation	+	+	±	+	+	+
Nurse	+	+	±	+	?	+
Home care	+	+	±	+	?	+
Emergency room	−	−	±	+	+	+
Outpatient hospital	+	+	±	+	+	+
Hospitalization						
Number of days	+	+	−	+	+	+
Episodes of surgery	+	+	−	+	+	+
Number of non-surgical procedures	+	±	−	±	+	+
Laboratory tests	+	−	−	±	±	+
Imaging tests	+	=	+	+	+	+
Drugs						
Prescription	+	−	+	+	+	+
Non-prescription	±	−	+	+	+	+
Rehabilitation services						
Physical therapy	+	−	±	+	+	+
Occupational therapy	+	−	−	+	+	+

Table 14 (*Continued*)

Indicator relevant for:	Conditions					
	Rheumatoid arthritis	Osteo-arthritis	Osteoporosis	Osteoporosis with fracture	Back pain and other spinal disorders	Major limb trauma
Durable medical equipment	–	–	–	+	±	+
Environmental adaptations						
Home alterations	+	+	–	+	?	+
Adaptations						
Work	+	+	–	+	+	+
Transport	+	+	–	+	+	+
Change of living status						
Nursing home	+	+	–	+	±	+
Other proposed indicators						
Primary care contact	+	+	±	+		
Falls			+	+		
Alternative treatments	+		+	+		
Returning to work					±	
Legal compensation	+				+	
Job change					+	
Socioeconomic group					+	
Educational level					+ and –	

+, highly relevant; ±, possibly relevant or less important; –, not relevant; ?, unknown.

[a] This list of indicators for measuring risk and the impact of the conditions could be used at various times to monitor change in the impact of musculoskeletal conditions during the Bone and Joint Decade and beyond. The list is broad and data may not be available from all populations; their availability and feasibility are considered separately in subsequent tables.

Table 15
Indicators of risk and impact in developed countries[a]

Indicator	Data available for the populations of these countries			Data not available for the populations of these countries but possible to collect		
	Most	Some	Few/none	Most	Some	Few/none
Risk factors						
Smoking	☒	☐	☐	☐	☐	☐
Alcohol	☒	☐	☐	☐	☐	☐
Body mass index	☒	☐	☐	☐	☐	☐
Family history	☐	☒	☐	☐	☐	☐
Heavy or repetitive activity	☐	☒	☐	☐	☒	☐
Impact						
Independence/disability						
Activities of daily living/ essential self-care	☒	☐	☐	☐	☒	☐
Complex activities of daily living/leisure activities	☐	☒	☐	☐	☒	☐
Quality of life						
Physical dimension	☒	☐	☐	☐	☒	☐
Mental dimension/ psychological well-being	☒	☐	☐	☐	☒	☐
Social dimension	☒	☐	☐	☐	☒	☐
Work loss						
Disability pension	☐	☒	☐	☐	☒	☐
Worker compensation	☐	☒	☐	☐	☒	☐
Mortality						
Related to condition or intervention	☒	☐	☐	☐	☐	☐
Resource utilization						
Number of visits						
Physician	☐	☒	☐	☐	☒	☐
Consultation	☐	☒	☐	☐	☒	☐
Nurse	☐	☐	☒	☐	☒	☐
Home care	☐	☒	☐	☐	☒	☐
Emergency room	☐	☒	☐	☐	☒	☐
Outpatient hospital	☐	☒	☐	☐	☒	☐
Hospitalization						
Number of days	☒	☐	☐	☐	☒	☐
Episodes of surgery	☐	☒	☐	☐	☒	☐
Number of non-surgical procedures	☐	☒	☐	☐	☒	☐
Laboratory tests	☐	☒	☐	☐	☐	☒
Imaging tests	☒	☐	☐	☐	☐	☒
Drugs						
Prescription	☒	☐	☐	☐	☒	☐
Non-prescription	☒	☐	☐	☐	☒	☐

Table 15 *(Continued)*

Indicator	Data available for the populations of these countries			Data not available for the populations of these countries but possible to collect		
	Most	Some	Few/none	Most	Some	Few/none
Rehabilitation services						
Physical therapy	☐	☒	☐	☐	☐	☒
Occupational therapy	☐	☒	☐	☐	☐	☒
Durable medical equipment	☐	☐	☒	☐	☐	☒
Environmental adaptations						
Home alterations	☐	☐	☒	☐	☐	☒
Adaptations:						
Work	☐	☐	☒	☐	☐	☒
Transport	☐	☐	☒	☐	☐	☒
Change of living status						
Nursing home	☐	☒	☐	☐	☐	☐
Other appropriate indicators						
Comorbidity	☐	☐	☒	☐	☒	☐
Primary care costs	☐	☐	☒	☐	☒	☐
Specialist costs	☐	☐	☒	☐	☒	☐
Educational level	☐	☐	☒	☐	☒	☐

[a] The availability of data for various non-instrument indicators that can be related to musculoskeletal conditions as a whole or to a specific condition, and the feasibility of collecting the data. The results are expressed as the proportion of countries that responded.

Table 16

Indicators of risk and impact in developing countries[a]

Indicator	Data available for the populations of these countries			Data not available for the populations of these countries but possible to collect		
	Most	Some	Few/none	Most	Some	Few/none
Risk factors						
Smoking	☐	☐	☒	☐	☐	☐
Alcohol	☐	☐	☒	☐	☐	☐
Body mass index	☐	☐	☒	☐	☐	☒
Family history	☐	☐	☒	☐	☐	☐
Impact						
Independence/disability						
Activities of daily living/ essential self-care	☐	☐	☒	☐	☐	☐
Complex activities of daily living/leisure activities	☐	☐	☒	☐	☐	☒
Quality of life						
Physical dimension	☐	☒	☐	☐	☐	☐
Mental dimension/ psychological well-being	☐	☐	☒	☐	☐	☒

Table 16 (*Continued*)

Indicator	Data available for the populations of these countries			Data not available for the populations of these countries but possible to collect		
	Most	Some	Few/none	Most	Some	Few/none
Social dimension	☐	☐	☒	☐	☐	☒
Work loss						
Disability pension	☐	☐	☒	☐	☐	☒
Worker compensation	☐	☐	☒	☐	☐	☒
Mortality						
Related to condition or intervention	☐	☐	☒	☐	☐	☒
Resource utilization						
Number of visits						
Physician	☐	☐	☒	☐	☒	☐
Consultation	☐	☐	☒	☐	☒	☐
Nurse	☐	☐	☐	☐	☒	☐
Home care	☐	☐	☐	☐	☒	☐
Emergency room	☐	☐	☐	☐	☒	☐
Outpatient hospital	☐	☐	☒	☐	☒	☐
Hospitalization						
Number of days	☐	☐	☒	☐	☐	☒
Episodes of surgery	☐	☐	☒	☐	☐	☒
Number of nonsurgical procedures	☐	☐	☐	☐	☐	☒
Laboratory tests	☐	☒	☐	☐	☐	☒
Imaging tests	☐	☐	☒	☐	☐	☒
Drugs						
Prescription	☐	☒	☐	☐	☐	☒
Nonprescription	☐	☒	☐	☐	☐	☒
Rehabilitation services						
Physical therapy	☐	☒	☐	☐	☐	☒
Occupational therapy	☐	☒	☐	☐	☐	☒
Durable medical equipment	☐	☐	☐	☐	☐	☒
Environmental adaptations						
Home alterations	☐	☐	☒	☐	☐	☒
Adaptations						
Work	☐	☐	☒	☐	☐	☒
Transport	☐	☐	☒	☐	☐	☒
Change of living status						
Nursing home	☐	☐	☐	☐	☐	☒
Other appropriate indicators						
Employability changes	☐	☐	☐	☐	☐	☐
Traditional medicines and treatments	☐	☐	☐	☐	☐	☐

[a] The availability of data for various non-instrument indicators that can be related to musculoskeletal conditions as a whole or to a specific condition, and the feasibility of collecting the data. The results are expressed as the proportion of countries that responded.

used at various times during the Bone and Joint Decade to monitor change in the health burden. Some factors place individuals at risk of injury or of developing a disease. The common risk factors of smoking, alcohol consumption, BMI and family history are included here.

A musculoskeletal condition or injury may affect a person's ability to remain independent in daily life or to work. Although individuals may be able to function independently, their health-related quality of life may be influenced in physical, emotional or social terms. An individual's employment may also be affected. In this connection the possibilities range from complete incapacity for work to adaptation to the regular work environment. Between these extremes there may be modified responsibilities or time commitments.

Musculoskeletal conditions impinge on the health care system in relation to hospitals, rehabilitation or nursing care facilities, services, equipment, personnel, laboratory and imaging tests, and prescription drugs. In certain circumstances, adaptations to the environment, either at work or at home, may be necessary in order to accommodate an individual with a musculoskeletal disease or injury.

Of interest to many countries and economies is an estimate of the cost of musculoskeletal conditions in economic terms. One frequently used way of examining the cost of health care is to divide it into direct, indirect and intangible categories. Hospitalization days, for example, can be assigned a monetary value, this being an example of a direct cost. Indirect costs, such as those for transportation to the place of treatment, add to the overall burden. Most difficult to assess, and not included here as an indicator, is the intangible cost of pain and suffering. These economic indicators give another dimension to the measurement of the burden of disease.

6.2 Rheumatoid arthritis

6.2.1 *Health indicators*

Indicators that can be used to measure the risk or health impact of rheumatoid arthritis and to monitor changes in the disease have been reviewed.

Risk factors

Risk factors for rheumatoid arthritis include gender, a family history of rheumatoid arthritis, and specific human leukocyte antigen (HLA) alleles. However, these factors are not at work in all populations. The HLA *DRB1* allele has been associated with the severity of rheumatoid arthritis in Anglo-Saxon populations but not in populations in the Mediterranean area (*138*). This geographical variation clearly hinders international comparisons. An attempt should be made to evaluate smoking, high BMI, previous blood transfusion and other possible risk factors in different populations.

Impact

The impact of rheumatoid arthritis is reflected by the effect of the disease on both simple and complex activities of daily living as well as by its broad effects on the different dimensions of the quality of life (Section 4). Work capacity is affected in most individuals within five years.

Resource utilization

In most countries, people with rheumatoid arthritis receive continuous health care, at least part of it in a secondary care setting. They often require adaptations to their workplace and home, as well as social support. Indicators that can be used to document the utilization of resources include the number of visits to outpatient clinics, hospital admissions, deaths, laboratory and imaging procedures, and the number and types of treatment and environmental adaptation. The relative importance of these indicators differs greatly according to the duration and severity of the rheumatoid arthritis.

One of the health indicators routinely collected in many developed countries is that of mortality. However, its relationship with rheumatoid arthritis is not easy to establish. Indeed, more than half the death certificates of patients who had rheumatoid arthritis fail to mention the disease. Mortality could also be registered in developing countries, allowing international comparisons. The long-term survival of patients with rheumatoid arthritis is reduced, particularly in women. A recent study from Norway confirmed a significant rise in mortality among females with rheumatoid arthritis because of cardiovascular disease (*139*). Mortality is generally lower in population-based studies of rheumatoid arthritis than in studies of patients in the clinical setting, where a more severe form of the disease is usually encountered.

Mortality is related to the severity of rheumatoid arthritis as expressed by functional status, health status, the perception of health status, radiological damage and extra-articular manifestations. Comorbidity, formal education, and socioeconomic and marital status may affect survival, but race has no bearing on this. In general, patients with rheumatoid arthritis die from the same causes as the general population but at an earlier age. In some studies a higher death rate has been found to arise from infection, renal disease, cardiovascular disease and malignancy among persons with rheumatoid arthritis than in the general population.

Problems associated with studies of mortality among people with rheumatoid arthritis relate to the classification of patients with non-standardized criteria and the lack of the "rheumatoid arthritis" diagnosis on death certificates. In addition, the provision of treatment was, until recently, rarely considered to be a factor influencing mortality. It should now be taken into account, however, because more aggressive therapy can affect outcome.

6.2.2 *Economic indicators*

The economic burden of rheumatoid arthritis can be evaluated by considering cost. This can be divided into direct cost (treatment, social services and private expenditure), indirect cost (lost productivity, lost earnings and lost tax revenue) and intangible cost, i.e. reduced quality of life. Articles from different countries dealing with the first two aspects have recently been reviewed (*140*). However, the results are hardly comparable because of differences in patient populations, treatments and study methods (sample surveys versus national prevalence data). In addition, health systems change over time, rates of exchange fluctuate, and public and private financing varies. The concept of resource utilization, rather than its monetary equivalent, is more useful for quantifying the economic burden of rheumatoid arthritis. It would probably be better to consider three kinds of measures: natural units such as physician visits or work time lost, monetary cost expressed in local currencies, and monetary cost expressed in purchasing parity, i.e. how many items of a certain type can be bought with a unit of local currency.

Most of these indicators cannot be used in developing countries because their health systems are not organized in the same way as those in developed countries. In the USA, most of the cost of rheumatoid arthritis has been shifted to outpatient care and drug treatment because patients with this disease are not admitted to hospital unless there is a severe complication or a need for surgery. Moreover, the economic value of lost productivity differs from country to country in relation to the overall employment rate (especially among women), the wage level and expected social roles. There is a need for a simple indicator that could be universally used. The mortality rate and the number of hospital visits might be good candidates for the evaluation of the impact of rheumatoid arthritis.

6.3 Osteoarthritis

6.3.1 *Health indicators*

Risk factors

The four main risk factors for osteoarthritis are age (the condition being more common in older people), family history, obesity and any form of joint trauma. Trauma predisposing to osteoarthritis may be related to repetitive activities rather than to a single event. There is consequently some association between certain types of osteoarthritis and certain occupations. Osteoarthritis of the knee, for example, is more common in persons with occupations involving heavy lifting and knee-bending activities than in members of the general population. In developed countries, osteoarthritis of the hip is more common in farmers than in persons engaged in other occupations. There are also racial differences in the apparent prevalence and expression of osteoarthritis at different joint sites, and there is evidence of some genetic predisposition. However, the problems encountered when defining osteoarthritis as a disease entity, outlined in Section 3, make international comparisons difficult.

Impact

Pain or discomfort, limitation of activity and reduced participation are the main recognized outcomes and health indicators associated with osteoarthritis. Data on these indicators can easily be collected in most countries through the adaptation of self-report instruments.

Resource utilization

Very little is known about this area, which concerns a highly variable set of symptoms in older people, i.e. pain and stiffness in joints and difficulty with certain activities. Many of these people have comorbidities, and many regard such symptoms as an inevitable part of ageing. However, in some countries, such as the USA, survey data suggest that this complex is so common, and that enough people are so intolerant of the symptoms, that resource use is massively greater than for any other recognizable musculoskeletal problem (Section 5).

6.3.2 *Economic indicators*

Economic indicators present a problem in osteoarthritis because the most relevant data to collect relate to the use of medical resources, for instance in connection with total hip replacement. This depends more on cultural, economic and health care provision issues in countries than on the condition itself. Lost work can be recorded, but the major impact of osteoarthritis is on people older than working age.

The Australian Institute of Health and Welfare estimated that the total health system cost of osteoarthritis in Australia was AUS$ 624.0 million in 1993–1994, approximately 21% of the total expenditure on musculoskeletal disorders (*81*). Of the total cost, 12.8% was contained within the medical services (general practitioners and specialists) and approximately 9% within the pharmaceutical sector (prescription and over-the-counter expenditure); AUS$ 35.9 million was spent within the field of allied health on osteoarthritis (5.8%), very close to the total expenditure on osteoarthritis in general practice (AUS$ 35.8 million). Under 1% of the total expenditure on osteoarthritis was spent on research (AUS$ 5.4 million). The hospital cost of osteoarthritis was spread quite evenly between public and private institutions (AUS$ 131.7 million and AUS$ 134.8 million respectively). The total hospital cost for osteoarthritis amounted to 42.7% of the total expenditure on osteoarthritis. It is reasonable to assume that most hospital expenditure results from joint replacements and ancillary costs associated with these procedures.

In 1997–1998 the average costs of hip replacement for public hospitals in Australia with and without complications were AUS$ 12275 and AUS$ 10412 respectively (*141*). These costs included all the ancillary services provided during the procedure. It can be estimated from this that the total costs for hip replacement in all Australian hospitals ($n = 21\,402$) were between AUS$ 223 million and AUS$ 263 million (the average costs for all complications and no complications respectively). Economic burden, as measured by hospital statistics, is a crude measure of the true cost of osteoarthritis because a significant proportion of cases are never treated within the hospital system.

March et al. (personal communication, 1999) conducted a prospective cohort study in Australia of 70 patients with osteoarthritis in order to determine the cost and social aspects relating to illness within the community. Patients were required to complete detailed cost diaries for a 12-month period, listing every cost relating to their arthritis under each type of expenditure heading. The range of expenditure that patients incurred in relation to their osteoarthritis ranged from zero to over AUS$ 2000. As expected, expenditure directly related to osteoarthritis increased as the duration of arthritis increased and physical function declined. Unexpectedly, however, females tended to spend more than males on their osteoarthritis, despite a similar health status.

6.4 Osteoporosis

6.4.1 *Health indicators*

Risk factors

Risk factors for a low BMD include age, female sex, early menopause, low body weight, immobility, smoking, alcohol abuse, corticosteroid use and thyrotoxicosis.

Risk factors for hip fracture include age, female sex, family history (maternal hip fracture), previous fracture (after the age of 50 years), low body weight, a low mobility and low activity level, visual disturbance, corticosteroid use, thyrotoxicosis, the use of long-acting benzodiazepines, the use of antiepileptics and a low calcium intake (*142*, *143*). Risk factors for vertebral fracture include age, female sex, a previous distal forearm or vertebral fracture, low body weight and corticosteroid use (*144*, *145*). It should be noted that the risk factors for hip fracture include those for falls (low activity, benzodiazepine and antiepileptic usage, and immobility). Patients with hip fractures and those with three or more vertebral fractures usually show some comorbidity.

The assessment of BMD is essential for the diagnosis of osteoporosis in its preclinical stage (stage 1). BMD is usually assessed by DXA. DXA equipment is widely but unevenly available in developed countries. The cross-calibration of DXA machines is not perfect, and different types use different reference values (*146*). Consequently, a patient may be diagnosed as osteoporotic in one centre but osteopenic or even normal in another. The site of measurement may also have a bearing on such results.

Impact

Quality of life issues have previously been mentioned (Section 4). They relate to the site of fracture, pain chronicity and impairment of function. Work loss, disability pension and worker compensation are not always of relevance in view of the age at which most osteoporotic fractures happen. Most hip fractures occur after the age of 75 years. Distal radius fractures and vertebral fractures do, however, have a significant impact, possibly resulting in work loss and its financial consequences. This needs to be calculated. Hip fractures are associated with an excess mortality of 20% during the first year after fracture. Vertebral fractures are associated with an excess mortality of about 5% in 5 years (*93*).

Resource utilization

Resource utilization is another important indicator, e.g. consultation with physicians and the use of facilities associated with nurses, home carers, emergency rooms and outpatient departments. Hospitalization is currently the best documented aspect of resource utilization in most countries, particularly developed countries. The available data include the numbers of days spent in hospital and the numbers of surgical and non-surgical procedures. Almost all patients with hip fracture in developed countries are admitted to hospital and undergo surgery, many requiring extensive rehabilitation in special units or nursing homes. About 25–30% of patients require permanent care in a nursing home after discharge from hospital. About 10% of patients with an acute vertebral fracture are admitted to hospital, and 5–10% of those with distal radius fracture are admitted to hospital for a short time.

Diagnostic tests, such as BMD, form the basis of diagnosis. The measurement of BMD is comparable to measuring blood pressure for the prediction of stroke and is substantially better than measuring serum cholesterol as a means of predicting cardiovascular disease. Equipment for measuring BMD, however, is unevenly distributed. It is mainly available in developed countries, but even there it is not uniformly available. Laboratory tests are important but are less commonly performed.

Other important indicators of utilization are medications (whether or not they are prescribed), rehabilitation services providing physical and occupational therapy, walking aids and rollators, and environmental adaptations in the home, on transport and elsewhere (*147*). Change of residence is a highly important indicator, e.g. from a house or apartment to a nursing home or rest home.

Emphasis must be placed on risk indicators, including previous fracture, family history, low body weight, immobility and the risk of falling. Patients with risk factors should be referred for BMD measurement (case-finding). However, the screening of populations by BMD measurement is not recommended.

6.4.2 *Economic indicators*

All the indicators that are recommended as being important can be converted into monetary terms. Data on the costs of hip fracture during the first and subsequent years after the incident are available (*148*). Cost calculations have also been made for vertebral fractures. Several economic models are used in developed countries in order to calculate the effect of interventions in osteoporosis, some of them having been published (*149*). Until recently the majority of studies in this field examined the cost-effectiveness of intervention with estrogen, usually targeted at the menopause (*150*), but such assessments are complicated by the extraskeletal risks and benefits of hormone replacement treatment. More recently, health economics has begun to focus on interventions targeted specifically at skeletal disease (*149*).

The following recommendations can be made.

- Every hospital should record all patients with hip fracture according to age and sex, so that adequate worldwide statistics on the subject can be acquired.

- A single representative national registration system for hip fractures should be established in every country.
- If possible, statistics should indicate the length of hospital stay, the operation performed, mortality, admission to a rehabilitation centre or nursing home after hip fracture, and an estimate of the direct and indirect costs.
- Hospital admission rates for other osteoporotic fractures should be assessed.
- Utility data should be obtained for hip and vertebral fractures, with reference to the societal and patient perspectives.
- The burden of osteoporotic fractures (hip fractures and all other osteoporotic fractures) should be compared with the burdens of other noncommunicable diseases, such as diabetes and breast cancer.
- The capacity for current BMD measurement and the projected need for it should be assessed in every country.
- BMD measurements should be better standardized so that every patient can be consistently classified as normal, osteopenic or osteoporotic in different centres.
- An assessment of risk for hip and other osteoporotic fractures involving a consideration of risk factors (±BMD) should replace the measurement of BMD alone.

6.5 Spinal disorders

The societal and individual impact of spinal disorders may be measured by using health and economic indicators to reflect the utilization of global resources. Unfortunately, important epidemiological data are missing in large areas of the world, without which the natural course of nonspecific spinal disorders and factors influencing their development and cost cannot be fully determined. Agreement on definitions, classification and staging is required. In addition, methods are required for separating the problem of back pain from that of disability caused by nonspecific spinal disorders.

6.5.1 *Health indicators*

Risk factors

Recent studies (*111*, *112*) blame various risk factors for the increased incidence of nonspecific musculoskeletal spinal disorders (see Table 11). A detailed analysis of musculoskeletal disorders in the workplace has led to the conclusion that there is a moderate to strong association between nonspecific spinal disorders and heavy physical loading. In respect of low back pain the physical parameters include the manual handling of material, load moment, frequent bending and twisting, heavy physical work and whole-body vibration (*151–155*). For the cervical spine the most common risk factors are exposure to repetitive movement of the neck and arm or arms, a static posture and segmental vibration exposure through hand-held tools (*69*, *156*).

In general there is a weak positive association between increased height and disc herniation (*157*, *158*). Obesity, regardless of height, is associated with disc degeneration and low back pain (*159*, *160*). Although large, tall people are likely to place a greater load on their intervertebral discs than other people, they are also likely to have larger discs (*161*). That these people may have to live and work in relatively awkward positions because of their size is probably a more plausible explanation of their predicament (*162*).

A genetic factor may influence spinal disorders involving the intervertebral discs. Studies show a positive family history as a risk factor for disc herniation (*163*). The exact cause of this genetic predisposition is not known. It could be the result of congenital spinal abnormalities (*164*) or a small vertebral canal (*165*), which would increase sensitivity to pressure on the nerve root. Further studies are needed in this area.

Work-related psychosocial factors associated with spinal disorders include a rapid work rate, monotonous work, low job satisfaction, a low decision latitude and job stress. Other characteristics affecting susceptibility to spinal disorders include age, gender, BMI and individual psychosocial factors (*69*, *96*, *152*, *166*, *167*).

Impact

Indicators that may be used to measure the health impact of specific and nonspecific spinal disorders and to monitor changes in the diseases are pain, limitation of activities and limitation of participation. Data on these indicators may easily be collected in most countries through the adaptation of self-report instruments. The most important domains, in rank order, were considered to be those shown in Table 17. The principal covariates were age, gender and comorbidity. The impact of spinal disorders on the quality of life increases with age and is greater in males than in females. It also increases with the recurrence and duration of episodes.

The following are additional items to consider when measuring the health impact of nonspecific musculoskeletal spinal disorders and monitoring changes in the diseases.

Mortality. Mortality is a limited indicator or outcome for spinal disorders, although issues of comorbidity need further study.

Table 17
Health indicators for specific and nonspecific spinal disorders in rank order

Specific spinal disorders	Nonspecific spinal disorders
Limitation of physical activity	Pain
Restricted participation (handicap)	Limitation of physical activity
Pain	Restricted participation (handicap)
Mobility/ambulation	Mobility/ambulation
Self-care	Self-care
Social activities/roles	Social activities/roles

Morbidity. In most epidemiological studies the prevalence of present or past back pain has been assessed by means of interviews or questionnaires that have used complex wording and have included implicit grading schemes and/or exclusions. It is highly recommended that simple questions and explicit grading schemes be used instead. A simple system might use actual pain intensity (on a numerical rating scale of 0–10), a questionnaire on activities of daily living/function, and a tool for recording the duration of episodes. Additional data may be obtained on temporal and course-related variables.

Other information related to back pain. Previous back pain (in the last week, month, year or ever), the duration of the current episode, the number of days and/or episodes of back pain during the past 12 months and the topography of the pain, i.e. the location and size of the painful area, and any radiation of the pain, should be noted. "Only occurrence" is routinely recorded. More data are collected in some countries, often in a highly idiosyncratic manner. It would be easy to elicit further data, at least for grading purposes.

Other morbidity characteristics. Functional losses may be determined by evaluating the subcategories of functional capacity, such as mobility (part of the activities of daily living [ADL]), transportation, leisure activities, sexual activities and other social role handicaps (occupation and household). The concept of amplification is important in nonspecific spinal disorders because it implies that in cases of back pain there are usually also complaints about other pain, other bodily complaints (somatization), psychological distress (depression or anxiety), impaired cognition and dysfunctional pain behaviour. Additional characteristics include limitations in the individual's major role and limitations in social and recreational activities.

Impact on other family members. There may be a limitation of family activities, parenting and other social consequences, as well as an effect on participation as a family in several of the other subcategories.

6.5.2 *Economic indicators*

The economic burden of spinal disorders may be evaluated by considering costs. These may be divided into:

- — direct costs (medical expenditure, such as the cost of prevention, detection, treatment, rehabilitation, long-term care and ongoing medical and private expenditure);
- — indirect costs (lost work output attributable to a reduced capacity for activity, such as lost productivity, lost earnings, lost opportunities for family members, lost earnings of family members and lost tax revenue);
- — intangible costs (psychosocial burden resulting in reduced quality of life, such as job stress, economic stress, family stress and suffering).

Reports dealing with direct and indirect costs from different countries have recently been reviewed and discussed (*168–170*). The results are hardly comparable, however, because of differences in patient populations, treatments and study methods (e.g. sample surveys versus national prevalence data). Work disability caused by back pain is often routinely recorded but is not comparable between different social security systems. Moreover, health systems change over time, rates of exchange fluctuate, and public and private financing varies.

The concept of resource utilization, rather than its monetary equivalent, is more useful for quantifying the economic burden of spinal disorders, although it too is subject to various sociocultural influences. Indicators that may be used to evaluate resource utilization include the number of visits to outpatient clinics, hospital admissions, mortality, laboratory and imaging procedures, medical management, environmental adaptations, and single or complex rehabilitation services such as physical therapy, occupational therapy and durable medical equipment. The relative importance of these indicators differs greatly according to the duration of spinal disorders and their severity. Many of them cannot be used in developing countries because of variations in the organization of health systems. There is thus a need to reach agreement on simple indicators that could be used universally.

Data exist on the economic consequences of work loss caused by nonspecific musculoskeletal spinal disorders in developed countries. In the USA the tangible expenditure (i.e. medical care and indemnity payments) and the intangible costs (i.e. production loss, employee retraining, increased consumer cost and litigation) associated with spinal disorders currently totals over US$ 50 billion (*61*, *69*, *171*).

Although comparative impact data for spinal disorders are not universally available, statistics on prevalence, impact and resource utilization are included here so as to emphasize the magnitude of the problem in the USA (Tables 18 and 19). These statistics are derived from the National Health Interview Survey conducted by the National Center for Health Statistics, the American Hospital Association Hospital Survey and other health needs collection instruments in 1996. The data were analysed and provided by the American Academy of Orthopaedic Surgeons.

Musculoskeletal disorders are the most frequent cause of physical disability, at least in developed countries (*172*). Mortality attributable to infectious diseases is decreasing, and the global population is ageing. The prevalence of many musculoskeletal disorders increases with age, and consequently there is likely to be an increasing number of people with chronic disabling disorders of this kind. The potential impact of this on needs for health care and community support is enormous.

6.6 Severe limb trauma

6.6.1 *Health indicators*

Risk factors

Factors that increase the risk of sustaining a limb trauma vary with the etiology or external cause of the injury, e.g. a fall, road traffic accident or assault. In order to reduce the overall impact of severe limb trauma, a surveillance of these risk factors is needed so that opportunities for intervention can be identified (*173*).

The risk of falls and the associated limb injury is greatest among the elderly. In the USA, one in three people over the age of 65 years falls each year. Of these, one-quarter are injured and another quarter restrict their activities for fear of another fall. Risk factors for falls among the elderly include those related to the host (e.g. visual, cognitive, neurological and physical impairments) and environmental hazards (loose rugs, ice and slippery surfaces, uneven floors and poor lighting). The risk of falling increases linearly with the number of risk factors present (*174*).

Adolescents and young adults are, on the other hand, typically at highest risk of limb injury resulting from road traffic accidents. Major factors contributing to the likelihood of this kind of accident include speed, vehicle instability, braking deficiencies, inadequate road design and alcoholic intoxication. Once an accident has occurred, the determinants of the extent and severity of injury include the speed of

Table 18

Back pain[a] in the general population of the USA, 1996

	Age group (years)										
	0–4	5–14	15–24	25–34	35–44	45–54	55–64	65–74	75–84	85+	Total
Number of cases											
Males	—	—	220 000	398 000	1 104 000	1 449 000	899 000	783 000	335 000	86 000[b]	5 274 000
Females	—	—	274 000	481 000	696 000	1 684 000	1 286 000	1 025 000	681 000	94 000[b]	6 221 000
Total	—	—	494 000	879 000	1 800 000	3 133 000	2 185 000	1 808 000	1 016 000	180 000[b]	11 495 000
Prevalence per 100 000 persons											
Males	—	—	12 100	20 100	52 100	92 500	89 900	95 200	80 100	94 000	40 900
Females	—	—	15 200	23 500	31 800	102 200	116 900	100 700	107 400	48 900	45 900
Total	—	—	13 700	21 800	41 800	97 500	104 000	98 300	96 600	63 400	43 500

[a] International Classification of Diseases-9 codes 720, 721.2–721.9, 724, 722.1–722.2, 722.3, 722.5–722.6, 722.70–722.72, 722.80, 722.82–722.83, 722.90, 22.92–722.93

[b] Data may not be statistically reliable because of a limited sample size.

Table 19

Non-instrument indices of the impact of back pain/injury in the USA, 1996

	Age Group (years)										
	0–4	5–14	15–24	25–34	35–44	45–54	55–64	65–74	75–84	85+	Total
Males											
Restricted activity days (1000s)	—	—	28 599	3655[c]	19 277	49 579	1 743[a]	17 326	576[a]	0	120 755
Bed days (1000s)	—	—	—	—	3 731[a]	3 779[a]	499[a]	—	—	0	8 009
Females											
Restricted activity days (1000s)	—	—	—	16 382	18 190	38 026	68 970	12 299	9 869	0	163 736
Bed days (1000s)		—	—	5 614[a]	4 970[a]	10 593	22 630	—	1 729[a]	0	45 536
Total											
Restricted activity days (1000s)	—	—	28 599	20 037	37 467	87 605	70 713	29 625	10 445	0	284 491
Bed days (1000s)	—	—	—	5 614[a]	8 701	14 372	23 129	—	1 729[a]	0	53 545

[a] Data may not be statistically reliable because of a limited sample size.

impact, the degree to which the vehicle involved can absorb the crash, and the use of safety devices and restraints (*175*).

Impact

Important indicators for measuring the impact of severe limb trauma include:

- — deaths attributable to major limb traumas (this being relevant for the most severely damaged or mangled extremities);
- — morbidity and complications (both short-term and long-term), such as malunions, non-unions, infections, osteomyelitis and post-traumatic arthritis;
- — disfigurement, including the loss of a limb and significant scarring;
- — symptoms such as pain (and phantom pain for amputees), joint stiffness, swelling, numbness, muscle cramping and muscle fatigue;
- — residual impairment, incorporating reduced range of motion, reduced strength, reduced sensation and impaired gait;
- — limitations in performing the specific activities or tasks needed for everyday living (e.g. walking, climbing stairs, grasping and handling small objects);
- — limitations in major role function;
- — limitations in other facets of participation, e.g. social functioning and participation in recreational activities;
- — psychosocial impact, including post-traumatic stress disorder and depression.

Priority should be given to the development of data appropriate to the following five indicators:

1. the occurrence of significant complications following initial acute care (e.g. unplanned rehospitalizations for complications in the year following injury);
2. a standardized measure of pain;
3. a standardized measure of physical functioning, i.e. limitations on performing the specific tasks necessary for everyday living;
4. a return to usual major role activity and/or a measure of lost productivity days or of days on which it is necessary to reduce usual activities;
5. a standardized measure of overall psychosocial well-being.

An overall preference-based assessment of disability or health-related quality of life which would encompass many of these indicators would be particularly useful for evaluating the global impact of limb trauma.

Few, if any, of these measures are available on a routine basis for well-defined populations with limb trauma. The difficulty of obtaining these measures is especially pronounced in developing countries, where, however, the burden of death and disability from injury appears to be significantly higher than in developed countries. It was recommended that special emphasis be placed on developing efficient low-cost approaches for collecting uniform indicators of health which could be used in developing countries. Such approaches would necessarily concentrate on:

— improving the completeness and accuracy of vital statistics registries;
— developing better methods for the routine registration of hospital admissions and attendance at outpatient and emergency departments;
— improving the use of the ICD for coding the nature and external cause of injuries;
— compiling population-based data for all hospitals across provinces and nations.

Data derived from clinical follow-up could be utilized to assess the long-term functional status of injured patients. Simple measures of functional status could be applied retrospectively in settings where outpatient record-keeping is of satisfactory quality. Special studies would be needed for more detailed measures. It was emphasized, however, that all forms of health service data would be limited in the settings of many developing countries, especially the lower-income countries of Africa and Asia, because of low utilization. For the foreseeable future a sizeable proportion of injured persons would not seek or would not have access to formal medical services. Household surveys should therefore be carried out periodically in order to assess the true incidence of injury and its functional, social and economic consequences.

Resource utilization

The utilization of health care services is often used as an indicator of health impact. For severe limb trauma these services include those associated with the initial acute management of the injury, the treatment of any sequelae and complications, and rehabilitation. For the most severe injuries, resulting in extensive neurovascular damage and limb loss, the use of services may continue throughout life. The need for ongoing treatment and rehabilitation depends on the nature and severity of the injury as well as on predisposing characteristics of the individual, such as age and the presence of comorbidity. However, caution is needed in the use of this indicator because the utilization of services is affected, in large measure, by their availability and accessibility.

6.6.2 *Economic indicators*

Economic indicators are summarized below as direct costs, indirect costs and human costs.

The direct costs are those of:

— prehospital care (emergency medical services);
— initial acute care (emergency department, other outpatient facility or hospitalization), including facility costs and professional fees;
— ongoing medical and surgical care for both routine follow-up and the treatment of complications (both inpatient and outpatient);
— rehabilitation (inpatient and outpatient);
— skilled nursing/long-term care;
— mental health services (inpatient and outpatient);
— home health care;
— personal assistance;
— special aids and assistive devices;
— medication;
— housing, transportation and work;
— vocational rehabilitation or retraining;
— insurance administration.

The indirect costs include:

— lost earnings for the injured person as a result of premature death or disability, including losses caused by inability to return to a previous job;
— lost earnings of family members;
— the value of informal care given by family members;
— the loss of land and other property;
— decreased educational opportunities for children and many other effects that contribute to the perpetuation of poverty.

The human costs are:

— the monetary value of pain and suffering;
— indebtedness.

Most important to the overall magnitude of the costs associated with limb trauma are:

— the initial acute treatment;
— rehabilitation and long-term care;
— assistive devices and accommodation;
— lost productivity of the injured person;
— in developing countries, the loss of land and other assets, increasing the vulnerability of families to future economic hardship.

The Scientific Group recommended that standardized assessments be developed and routinely used at selected sites around the world in order to increase the effectiveness with which the economic costs of major limb traumas were monitored.

7 Describing health status and the consequences of illness or injury for the individual

7.1 Introduction

This section is about health status measures and the data that have been collected by using them. Health status measures are standardized descriptions of health states that are often presented as multidimensional profiles of health. They are distinct from classifications of morbidity, symptoms or mortality such as are found in the ICD. Under the ICD, for example, an individual at a certain stage of rheumatoid arthritis would be placed in a single classification. Instead, health status measures provide information on a variety of domains that represent health. Regardless of the condition, information is provided on each domain. This information can be professionally observed through clinical examinations or observations, laboratory assessments or some type of performance test, or they can be self-reported. Self-reporting can be done by the individual concerned or by a family member or carer.

7.1.1 *Uses of data collected*

Health status measures provide additional information on illness and wellness, often from the individual's perspective if he or she is reporting either to a lay interviewer or when meeting with a professional. Data collected through health status measures are used as outcome indicators for monitoring, evaluating and planning, particularly in clinical trials or technology assessment trials. They are increasingly used for monitoring the health of populations. Such data may highlight subpopulations that are heavily burdened by a particular disease or condition, or may relate to particular age or sex groups. They may also provide information for advocacy and health promotion activities, particularly where people are interested in matters at the positive end of the spectrum, e.g. fitness. However, it is important to develop a common way of describing health regardless of the specific disease or condition, covering a comprehensive set of domains that make up health.

7.1.2 *Multidimensional health concept*

A large number of instruments have been developed which measure health in various domains that are sometimes called dimensions, indicators or scales. Different dimensions from some of the most popular generic health status instruments are shown in Table 20. This table

Table 20

Domains included in some common health status indicators

Health domains	QWB 1970	McM 1976	SIP 1976	QLI 1981	NHP 1981	FSQ 1986	Duke 1990	SF-36 1992	WHO QOL 1996	EQ-5D 1999	WHO DAS 1999
Overall well-being											
General health				✔			✔	✔			
Perceived health							✔				
Change in health											
Physical health		✔					✔		✔		
Activities/roles	✔			✔				✔		✔	✔
Work			✔			✔					
Home			✔								
Recreation			✔								
Ambulation			✔								
Eating			✔								
Energy/vitality					✔			✔			
Mobility/fitness	✔		✔		✔	✔	✔	✔		✔	✔
Pain/discomfort					✔		✔	✔		✔	
Self-care			✔	✔		✔				✔	✔
Sleep/rest			✔		✔						

Social health		✔					✔		✔		
Activities/roles	✔					✔		✔			
Communication			✔								
Interaction			✔		✔	✔					✔
Support				✔							
Mental health						✔	✔	✔	✔		
Activities/roles								✔			
Alertness			✔								
Anxiety/depression							✔			✔	
Cognition										✔	✔
Emotional status		✔	✔		✔						
Outlook				✔							
Self-esteem							✔				
Handicap/participation					✔						✔
Environment									✔		

QWB, Quality of Well-Being; McM, McMaster Health Index Questionaire; SIP Sickness Impact Profile; QLI, Quality of Life Index; NHP, Nottingham Health Profile; FSQ, Functional Status Questionnaire; Duke, Duke Health Profile; SF-36, Short Form Health Status Survey; WHOQOL, World Health Organization Quality of Life; EQ-5D, EuroQol Instrument; WHODAS, World Health Organization Disability Assessment Schedule (for additional information on these instruments, see Table 32).

illustrates the alternative ways in which, for example, physical health can be described.

Few instruments use the same labels for domains or scales, or cover the same content with respect to the questions that make up each domain. The range of domains included across instruments reflects different operational approaches to defining and measuring health. The content covered in each domain varies: some instruments use the same domain label but include different questions. The breadth or depth of content covered in each domain also varies, some including items focusing on a specific function, such as eating, others encompassing those items that assess a range of complex functions and activities, such as understanding and interacting. The main point is that no single standard set of domains and questions is used to describe health, although this would facilitate the comparison of health status across populations or disease groups.

7.1.3 *Limitations of currently available measures*

There is no clear conceptual basis for how the currently available measures define health. This is apparent from the different domains included in different instruments, even though each instrument claims to measure the concept of health generically.

Standardized protocols are lacking not only for description and measurement but also for the interpretation and comparison of health. This is particularly problematic with regard to the comparison of health across populations as well as across different subgroups within populations, although there have been some developments in the past decade towards improving this situation. For instance, there is a limited reference of disease-specific averages from different domains of health to those of populations. It would be useful, for example, to be able to see an SF-36 profile of people with rheumatoid arthritis in a population, as well as an SF-36 profile reflecting the profile of the general population, based on a nationally representative survey.

The application of these instruments and the data sets currently encountered, including even those few instruments with data from a relatively large number of countries, is mainly restricted to industrialized countries.

There is a lack of guidelines on selecting from the wide range of instruments available, either generic or disease-specific. Although there is much literature on different instruments for bone and joint diseases, this is not the case for many other areas.

7.1.4 *Boundary between health and well-being*

The unclear boundary between health and well-being presents a conceptual problem if health is an aspect of well-being and there is a desire to measure health. This problem translates into an operational challenge with respect to the items that we would want to include in health and those items of well-being that one considers important to health (Figure 16). Since one desires to compare health across different disease groups and populations, its definition has to be operationalized so that it can be measured and interpreted consistently.

There are several ways of cutting across this boundary. Indicators of health could be picked on the basis of there being a continuum from biological processes to well-being, otherwise termed the quality of life (Figure 17). Where the line would be drawn, or where indicators would be picked from, would be based on a normative process.

Another way of defining the boundary is to develop a model including the health state, its determinants and its consequences. This model could be included in some profile of health beyond those domains that actually describe the health state (Figure 18). One way of doing this would be to select indicators from data sources and to try to understand where they fit.

Figure 16
Boundary between health and non-health well-being

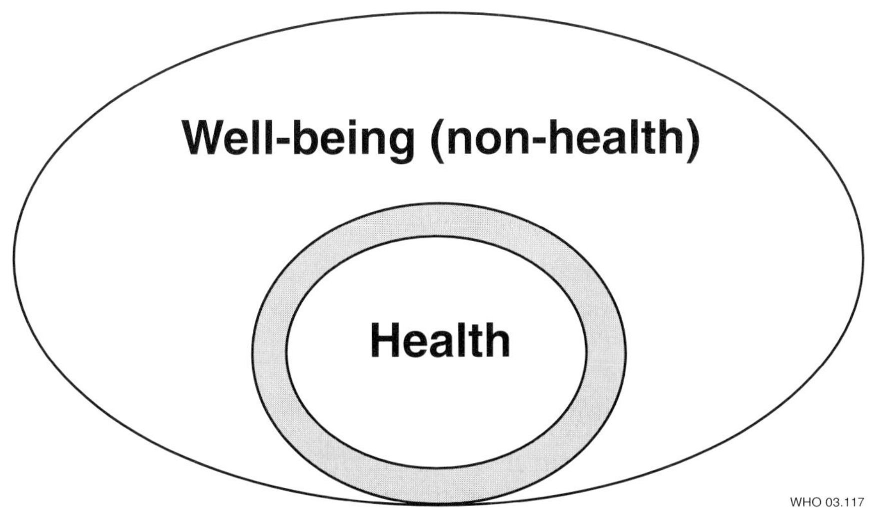

Figure 17
First model for alternative boundaries

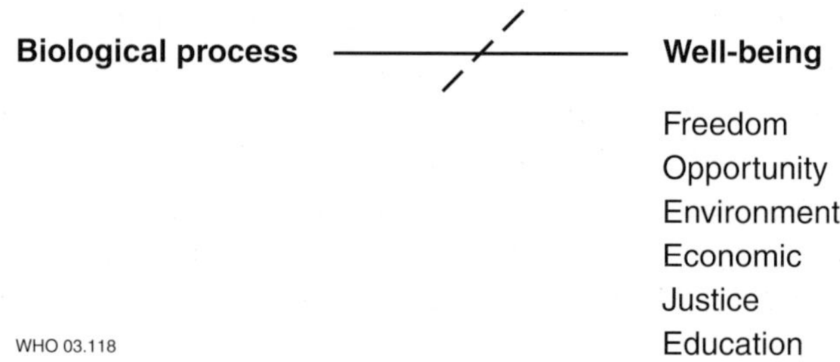

Figure 18
Second model for alternative boundaries

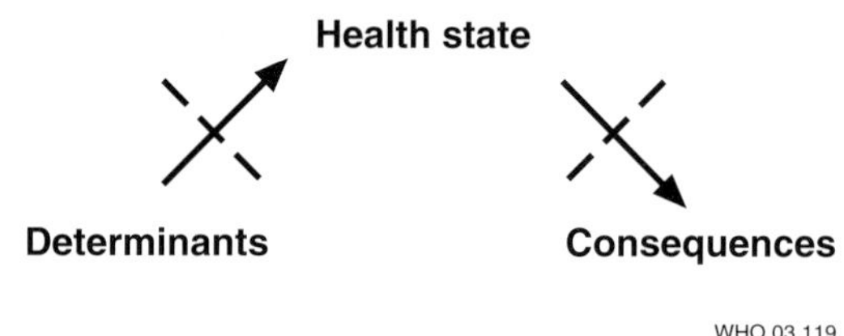

7.1.5 *Need for a common language and profile to describe health*

ICF may provide a way of helping to harmonize and compare existing measures and indicators of health. The revised classification considers body structures and body functions that are either organ or functionally based. Activity limitations include self-care, the ability to perform the usual activities, and the performance of other specific tasks. Many current instruments include domains or indicators from these two areas. However, the inclusion of domains in most instruments tends to be somewhat arbitrary. The third component of the revised ICF is restriction of participation, or handicap. Fewer measures of health status include indicators or domains that will map these areas.

Some instruments claim to measure "health-related quality of life" or "quality of life". An examination of the domains and items included, however, may reveal that the domains are, in most cases, precisely those that focus specifically on disability or other aspects of physical or cognitive functioning. It is therefore necessary to go to the domain level and review the items that are actually included before making a judgement about what an instrument measures.

Alternatively, certain domains may be too specific to structure or functions and may require specialized information that individuals are unable to self-report in a valid way. It may therefore be that self-reported information on activity limitations, participation or handicap is a better operational way of measuring the underlying health concept even if these are proxy measures of the health state. The HAQ was, for example, originally developed to provide information on five domains, but most of these related to physical disability. In the past few years, modifications have been suggested to include a broader range of domains capable of describing a wider range of problems, e.g. those related to advanced activities of daily living as well as psychological distress.

Another trend is to improve the ability to interpret scores. Information on how scores correlate with reduced fist closure, reduced hand spread, elevated platelet count or the presence of tender joints, in different age and sex groups, would, for example, help to explain the meaning of different scores based on self-reported assessments of health status.

7.1.6 *Description versus valuation of health*

In relation to Global Burden of Disease Studies it is important to distinguish between health status measurement and health state valuation. This distinction has been made by health economists and has a long history in the environmental field, where, for example, the description of good air quality is distinct from how much we value good air or polluted air.

Two summary measures of population health have been calculated within the Global Burden of Disease Studies, the DALY and the DALE (disability-adjusted life expectancy). Both combine information on the impact of premature death and of disability and other health outcomes. In order to calculate a DALY or a DALE, prevalence figures for different severity levels of disability and other aspects of health are required, either for each disease or for the population in general.

In order to construct either a DALY or a DALE, it is necessary to weight the time spent in different health states varying in severity from full or perfect health to almost death, in addition to using descriptive epidemiological data. This allows years of life lost from premature mortality to be combined with years spent in a health state worse than full health. All summary measures of population health require health state valuations as inputs. Likewise, cost-effectiveness analyses that measure the benefits of interventions in time-based units, e.g. QALYs, require health state valuations in order to assign weights to years spent in different states of health.

It is important to note the distinction between the measurement of health status along different domains of health and the valuation of different health states. Whereas different health status instruments may be used to describe health states, the purpose of health state valuations is to assign a single value to the time spent in different health states. This differs from the goal of health status measurement, which seeks to describe the current health of individuals in terms of multiple dimensions.

Once different disease stages of various bone and joint conditions have been clearly distinguished and agreement has been reached on how to describe health in a uniform way, it may be possible to undertake a valuation exercise. An example of how to describe an array of health states that are not specific to one particular disease is given by EuroQol, which describes health using the domains of self-care, usual activities, mobility and fitness, pain and discomfort, anxiety and depression, and cognition, with three levels of response, i.e. no problems, some problems and unable to perform.

The disease-specific approach to communicating a health state for valuation is to describe an individual with a particular disease at a particular stage and the level of health in terms of each of these six domains. The generic approach is to label the profile with numbers so as to distinguish severity levels, leaving out the disease label. Each method requires particular types of ability for analysis. Different disease states can be valued if they are described in a comparable way.

7.1.7 *Next steps*

The final aim of the workshop was to select indicators for monitoring bone and joint health over the following decade and to suggest core sets of domains to describe a complete health state. These core sets should be able to describe a broad range of health states that are not specific to any particular disease or condition but may be applicable and appropriate across populations. They should be parsimonious in including the smallest possible number of domains while trying to maximize the information being measured and communicated.

Domains that lend themselves to self-reporting should be considered if they are to be used for large-scale monitoring, e.g. through surveys. Self-reporting may, however, be affected by adaptation or coping with the disease or condition in question, or may be shaped by external factors that introduce differences in how people respond to a given level of health or inability to carry out a task. Approaches to adjusting for variations in how people self-report health status by age and sex, as well as by different disease groups and other social, cultural or economic aspects, are currently being investigated by WHO.

The selection of a core set of domains, the collection and analysis of existing health status data, and the standardization of methods for the future collection and analysis of data should lead to a clearer understanding of the current and future impact of musculoskeletal conditions on health.

7.2 Multidimensional approach to measuring health status for musculoskeletal conditions

Health status can be measured in many ways. The method employed may relate to the purpose for measuring health, the time available and the level of detail required. Using a single dimension (domain), a five-point scale (excellent, very good, good, fair or poor) represents a simple method. Other approaches provide a more detailed description by measuring more than one health domain and perhaps more than one attribute (subdomain) within a domain. The SF-36, for example, measures eight subdomains and represents health status by means of a multidimensional profile. An individual's level of performance is measured in each selected domain or subdomain. The set of scores across the domains is often called a health state.

Disease and injury conditions may not be static. Following injuries resulting from trauma, recovery progresses through a series of stages. Full recovery is reached if there is a return to normal health. For chronic disease, the progression through stages is in the opposite direction, from normal health to potentially severe disability or even death.

The experts in the disease or condition work groups conducted a measurement process that resulted in describing health states, categorized according to disease or injury stage. Each group selected from a common list the most important health domains that should be measured for the group's particular condition. The domains included physical health, social health, emotional health, etc., in which subdomains were nested, e.g. ambulation, pain and mobility. The selected domains, listed in order of perceived importance, formed the column headings in a table. A summary for all the conditions is given in Table 21.

For each subdomain the work groups assigned a performance rating using a scale that could be applied globally (e.g. a three-point rating scale in which 1 = performs with no difficulty, 2 = performs with some difficulty and 3 = cannot perform). This resulted in sets of scores or health states which formed the rows in the table. The health states were then grouped according to the disease stages that had been defined in an earlier working session. Table 22 shows a small sample of hypothetical health states for osteoarthritis.

Table 21

Summary of relevant domains and subdomains for musculoskeletal conditions

	Rheumatoid arthritis	Osteoarthritis Lower limb	Osteoarthritis Hand	Osteoporosis	Spinal disorders	Trauma Upper limb	Trauma Lower limb
Overall well-being	E						
General health	D			C			
Perceived health						A	A
Change in health	D					A	A
Physical health	A			A	X		
Activities/roles	a				X		
Work				c	X	A	A
Home				b		A	A
Recreation				b	X	A/B	A/B
Ambulation					X	A	A
Eating					X	A	C
Energy/vitality	a			d		B	B
Mobility/fitness				a	X	C	A
Pain/discomfort	a			a	X	A	A

Self-care	a	a		A	A
Sleep/rest		c		B	B
Social health	B	B	X		
Activities/roles	b	a	X		
Communication		c		A (writing)	C
Interaction	b	c		B	B
Support	b	b			
Mental health	C	D			
Activities/roles					
Alertness				C	C
Anxiety/depression	c	b	X	A	A
Cognition		d		C	C
Emotional status		b	X	A	A
Outlook		b		A	A
Self-esteem	c	b		A	A
Handicap/participation	D	B	X		
Environment					

A, most important domain; a, most important subdomain; X, applicable.

Table 22
Hypothetical health states for osteoarthritis

Disease Stage	Health domains			
	Physical		Social	Mental
	Mobility	Pain	Social role	Emotional status
Normal	1	1	1	1
I	1	2	1	1
	1	1	1	2
II	1	2	1	2
	2	1	1	2
III	2	2	2	2
	2	2	2	3
IV	2	3	3	3
	3	3	3	3

The most suitable instrument or instruments were identified to measure the different conditions that included, as far as possible, the health domains selected. These are described in the subsequent sections. They are also included in the inventory of published assessment instruments. The suitability of these selected instruments for global application was also considered.

7.3 Rheumatoid arthritis

7.3.1 *Health domains*

Rheumatoid arthritis affects body structure and functions in a number of ways, the extent of involvement depending on the severity of the disease and the effect of treatment. Patients' outcomes also depend on their ability to cope with their limitations. These are the result of the severity of the disease, comprising both the activity of the disease over time and the cumulative damage to the joints. At an early stage this impact may therefore be transient. It tends to become permanent and progressive in the later stages. The health domains of particular importance in rheumatoid arthritis were identified as follows (in decreasing order of importance) (Table 23):

1. physical health;
2. social health, including work roles and other activities;
3. mental health;
4. general health, change in health and handicap (considered by the panel to be equally important);
5. overall health.

The physical health domain includes:

Table 23

Rheumatoid arthritis: relevant domains and subdomains

	Relevant domains	Relevant subdomains	Normal	Rating scale by stages or categories of the condition							
				I		II		III		IV	
Overall well-being	E										
General health	D										
Perceived health											
Change in health	D										
Physical health	A										
Activities/roles		a	1	1	1	1	2	2	2	2	3
Work											
Home											
Recreation											
Ambulation											
Eating											
Energy/vitality		a	1	2	1	2	2	2	2	2	2
Mobility/fitness											
Pain/discomfort		a	1	2	1	2	2	2	2	3	3
Self-care		a	1								
Sleep/rest											

Table 23 (*Continued*)

	Relevant domains	Relevant subdomains	Normal	Rating scale by stages or categories of the condition							
				I		II		III		IV	
Social health	B										
Activities/roles		b	1	1	1	1	1	1	2	3	3
Communication											
Interaction		b	1	1	1	1	1	2	2	2	3
Support		b	1	1	1	1	1	2	2	2	3
Mental health	C										
Activities/roles											
Alertness											
Anxiety/depression		c	1	1	2	2	2	3	3	3	3
Cognition											
Emotional status											
Outlook											
Self-esteem		c	1	1	1	2	2	3	3	3	3
Handicap/participation	D										
Environment											
Additional domains proposed											
Sexuality	X										

A, most important domain; a, most important subdomain; 1, no impact; 2, mild impact; 3, moderate impact; 4, severe impact.

— physical function, such as activities of daily living and self-care;
— pain;
— energy/vitality, including fatigue and sleep disturbances.

Early morning stiffness, fatigability and non-restorative sleep are among the most important complaints of patients with rheumatoid arthritis of recent onset. An adjustment should be made for age.

The social health domain includes:

— activities/roles at work and at home or during recreation;
— interaction/isolation;
— support.

Limited communication in terms of impaired hearing or diminished visual acuity is probably not particularly important in rheumatoid arthritis. However, there are often limitations of communication through writing and mobility.

The mental health domain includes anxiety/depression and self-esteem/self-image.

Overall, the domains to be explored should include the core domains of physical function, pain, and social, psychological or emotional changes. In addition, it is important to consider body image, sexual activity, fatigue and employment.

7.3.2 *Possible health states*

Table 24 shows an example of hypothetical health states for rheumatoid arthritis. This table is, of course, an oversimplification of complex life experiences, which often show a fluctuation in opposite directions. It should also be remembered that the pace of deterioration in the different health domains at different disease stages is not synchronous. Rheumatoid arthritis is a chronic disease, and only some 10–20% of patients reach stable remission. Pain and stiffness are usually intense at the onset of the disease but can be transiently improved by successful treatment soon thereafter. In the later stages, mechanical pain, caused by subluxation and joint incongruity, adds to inflammatory pain. Anxiety is more evident in the early phases of rheumatoid arthritis, when patients are faced with an unexpected and unknown threat to their well-being, whereas depression becomes apparent in the chronic stage. Patients frequently adapt to the disease through changed working habits and expectations and the use of devices.

7.3.3 *Suggested instruments for measuring selected health domains*

There is no such thing as a perfect instrument that can capture the health domains thought to be most important in rheumatoid arthritis.

Table 24
Hypothetical health states for rheumatoid arthritis

Stage	Health domains							
	Physical			Social			Mental	
	ADL/SC	Pain	Energy/ vitality	Activity	Interaction	Support	Anxiety/ depression	Self-esteem/ self-image
Normal	1	1	1	1	1	1	1	1
I	1	2	2	1	1	1	1	1
	1	1	1	1	1	1	2	1
II	1	2	2	1	1	1	2	2
	2	2	2	1	1	1	2	2
III	2	2	2	2	2	2	3	3
	2	2	2	2	2	2	3	3
IV	2	3	2	3	2	2	3	3
	3	3	2	3	3	3	3	3

ADL/SC, activities of daily living/self-care.

However, the Arthritis Impact Measurement Scales-2 (AIMS-2), the Rheumatoid Arthritis Patient's Questionnaire and the SF-36 were provisionally identified as useful instruments that could address most of the important health domains.

7.4 Osteoarthritis

7.4.1 *Health domains*

Several domains were considered to be important in joint disorders (rheumatoid arthritis and osteoarthritis) (Table 25):

- Physical health: physical function, employment/work, pain, and fatigue.
- Social health: social function.
- Mental health: emotional function, self-image, sexuality.
- Handicap/participation.

The main recognized outcomes and health indicators associated with osteoarthritis are pain or discomfort, limitation of activities and restriction of participation. Data on these indicators can easily be collected in most countries through the adaptation of existing self-report instruments.

The most important attributes for lower limb osteoarthritis, in rank order, were considered to be:

— pain/discomfort;
— mobility;
— physical activities/roles;
— ambulation;
— restricted participation (handicap);
— social activities/roles.

Those for osteoarthritis of the hand, in rank order, were viewed as being:

— pain/discomfort;
— physical activities/roles;
— self-care;
— restricted participation (handicap);
— social activities/roles;
— eating.

7.4.2 *Possible health states*

This exercise could not be undertaken because it was not possible to agree on the different stages of osteoarthritis of the lower limb or hand.

Table 25
Osteoarthritis: relevant domains and subdomains

	Osteoarthritis of the lower limb		Osteoarthritis of the hand	
	Relevant domains	Relevant subdomains	Relevant domains	Relevant subdomains
Overall well-being				
General health				
Perceived health				
Change in health				
Physical health	A		A	
Activities/roles		c		b
Work				
Home				
Recreation				
Ambulation		d		
Eating				d
Energy/vitality				
Mobility/fitness		b		
Pain/discomfort		a		a
Self-care				c
Sleep/rest				
Social health	C		C	
Activities/roles		a		a
Communication				
Interaction				
Support				
Mental health				
Activities/roles				
Alertness				
Anxiety/depression				
Cognition				
Emotional status				
Outlook				
Self-esteem				
Handicap/participation	E		B	B
Environment				
Additional domains proposed				
Sexuality	X			

A, most important domain; a, most important subdomain.

7.4.3 ***Suggested instruments for measuring selected health domains***

The agreed instruments suitable for recording these domains are shown in Table 26. These instruments depend on self-reporting and therefore require a certain degree of literacy. They also need to be translated into the language and revalidated in the culture of the country in which they are used.

Table 26
Instruments for recording relevant domains in osteoarthritis

	Disease-specific	Generic
Lower limb	Western Ontario and McMaster Universities Osteoarthritis Index (WOMAC)	WHO Disability Assessment Schedule (WHODAS II)[a]
	Arthritis Impact Measurement Scales-2 (AIMS-2)[a]	Short Form Health Status Survey (SF-36)[a]
	Disease Repercussion Profile (DRP)[a]	
Upper limb	Australian/Canadian (AUSCAN) Osteoarthritis Hand Index	WHODAS II[a]
	Disabilites of the Arm, Shoulder and Hand (DASH) Outcome Measure	SF-36[a]
	DRP[a]	

[a] The Scientific Group had concern about the validity of these instruments for older people with osteoarthritis.

WOMAC has been designed to capture the essential elements of pain, stiffness and physical functioning in patients with osteoarthritis of the knee and/or hip joints. It has been translated into over 60 different languages and is most commonly used for self-reporting. It usually takes fewer than five minutes to complete. Other administration modes are possible, including the interviewer-delivered and telephone modes. WOMAC index is also available in both Likert and visual analogue scaled formats.

7.5 Osteoporosis

7.5.1 *Health domains*

Osteoporosis is characterized by a loss of bone mass with microarchitectural deterioration of the bone tissue and an increased risk of fracture, its clinical manifestation being fracture at a variety of skeletal sites. The health domains and their performance rating vary at different stages of the natural history of the disease. There may be little or no impact in the pre-fracture stage apart from that associated with any predisposing condition. Significant morbidity may occur immediately following fracture. Morbidity may then decrease among persons surviving into the chronic post-fracture stage (*176*).

The most important health domains for measuring the burden of osteoporosis are shown in Table 27. Pain with loss of physical function is the major outcome of any fracture (*26*, *87*). With more severe

Table 27
Health-related domains and subdomains relevant to osteoporosis

	Relevant domains	Relevant subdomains
General health	C	
Physical health	A	
Activities/roles		
Work		c
Home		b
Recreation		b
Ambulation		b
Eating		b
Energy/vitality		d
Mobility/fitness		a
Pain/discomfort		a
Self-care		a
Sleep/rest		c
Social health	B	
Activities/roles		a
Communication		c
Interaction		c
Support		b
Mental health	D	
Activities/roles		a
Alertness		d
Anxiety/depression		a
Cognition		d
Emotional status		b
Outlook		b
Self-esteem		a
Handicap/participation	B	

A, most important domain; a, most important subdomain.

fractures there are added social and mental consequences. Within the domain of physical function the subdomains of mobility and self-care are considered to be extremely important. The impact on activities and roles, followed by the need for support, is the most important of the social subdomains, although impairment of mobility and ambulation may have a major effect on communication and interaction. Mental health is affected not only by anxiety and depression but also by the changes in body shape and loss of self-esteem which accompany osteoporotic fractures, especially of the vertebrae.

7.5.2 *Possible health states*

In estimating the impact on quality of life, health states associated with osteoporotic fracture should be defined according to the fracture site and the time since the fracture occurred. This approach was used

Table 28

Impact on quality of life of various health states in osteoporotic patients

	Health domains				
	General	Pain	Physical	Social	Mental
Stage 1: Bone loss					
Bone loss (t < –2.5), no fractures	1	1	1	1	1
Stage 2: Fractures					
Colles' fracture					
acute (6 weeks)	2	3	3	3	1
late (1 year)	1	2	2	1	1
Vertebral fracture					
acute, clinical	3	4	3	3	3
late, clinical (1 year)	2	2	2	2	2
Crush fracture syndrome					
3 or more fractures, clinical (comorbidity)	4	4	4	4	4
Vertebral deformity					
one, radiological	1	1	2	1	1
multiple and/or severe deformities	3	3	3	3	3
Hip fractures					
Acute	4	4	4	4	4
chronic (1 year) independent	2	2	2	2	1
chronic (1 year) dependent, comorbidity	4	3	4	4	3
Other limb fracture					
Acute	2	3	3	3	1
chronic (1 year)	2	2	3	3	1
Fragility fractures in children					
mobility dependent	3	4	4	3	3
mobility independent	2	4	2	2	2

1, no impact; 2, mild impact; 3, moderate impact; 4, severe impact.

by the WHO Study Group (*1*) that assessed the impact (burden) of osteoporosis (Table 28). Ratings were assigned to different fractures for the various quality of life domains. The following key domains were considered: general health, pain, physical function, social function and mental function. Domains were rated as "no impact" (1), "mild impact" (2), "moderate impact" (3) or "severe impact" (4). The rationale for the various post-fracture health statuses was described in Section 4. Clinical vertebral fractures must be differentiated from radiographic vertebral deformities, which do not immediately come to clinical attention. Health states after hip fracture are classified as "chronic independent" in younger patients or "dependent", the latter being more common in elderly patients.

The most important covariates were age, gender and comorbidity. The impact of hip fracture on the quality of life increases with age and is greater in male patients than in female patients. The effect of vertebral fractures increases with their number and severity, as well as with age (*26*, *82*). Lumbar fractures have a greater impact on the quality of life than thoracic fractures (*26*).

Health status may considerably improve after the treatment of fracture, but data on changes in the quality of life are scarce (*176*). Some information is available on the quality of life during the first year following distal radius fracture: the total QALY loss amounted to about 2% (*91*). In contrast, vertebral fractures may cluster in individuals over a few years, leading to difficulty in characterizing a typical quality of life time-course (*82*, *83*, *92*).

A further problem relates to the various methodologies employed to obtain utility states, as different methods provide different values (*177*). The National Osteoporosis Foundation of the USA has provided utility values for all osteoporotic fractures on the basis of expert opinion (*178*). These need to be substantiated by empirical information. Nevertheless. they provide a mechanism for calculating the impact of different fractures on the total burden of osteoporosis (*40*). By means of the time trade-off method, utility data for hip fracture have been obtained from elderly women attending a fall clinic. They considered a hip fracture leading to nursing home admission to be a disaster with a utility of 0.15 (*179*).

7.5.3 *Suggested instruments for measuring selected health domains*

The following generic instruments have been used for quality of life assessment in osteoporotic patients: the NHP, SF-36 and EuroQol (EQ-5D). Two disease-specific, self-administered instruments for osteoporosis have been developed and validated: Qualeffo-41 and the OPAQ. Qualeffo-41, as well as the NHP and EQ-5D, shows a rising impact on the quality of life with an increasing number of vertebral fractures, the increase being greater for Qualeffo-41 than for either generic instrument (*26*). Qualeffo-41 scores also rise with an increasing number of incident vertebral fractures, indicating that this instrument is sensitive to change (*83*).

The best interviewer-based, disease-specific instrument is the OQLQ, which has been validated and subsequently condensed (*89*). An alternative is OPTQoL, which has also been validated (*90*). As generic instruments enable a comparison of the burden of osteoporosis with that of other diseases, it appears appropriate to use both a generic and a disease-specific questionnaire in future studies.

The Scientific Group concluded that a sufficient number of instruments were available for quality of life assessment among patients with osteoporosis.

7.5.4 *Issues relating to children*

Several issues merit attention in connection with osteoporosis in children. The definition of the disorder is problematic because of the variation in body size and its effect on BMD measurements by DXA. Osteoporosis in children may be defined with regard to the age-matched mean value (z-score <–2.5), although reference values are not widely available. There is a lack of information relating bone mass to fracture risk, but the condition can be staged as for adult disease. Osteoporosis sufferers can be divided into those without any impairment of mobility and those dependent on aids to mobility.

In considering body, person and society, it should be borne in mind that whereas the patient is a child, the affected unit is the family. Within health domains, applicability to the child/family unit is not considered, and specific problems of development and growth are not accounted for. The tools available have limited applicability: the Pediatric Evaluation of Disability Inventory has no age-standardized scores beyond the age of 7.5 years, and there is a need to acquire information on the Childhood Health Assessment Questionnaire.

The following recommendations can be made.

- Health stages should be better defined so that they can be used in clinical practice and the burden of disease can be calculated.
- Utility data should be obtained for all health states following an osteoporotic fracture.

7.6 Spinal disorders

7.6.1 *Health domains*

Health status was evaluated by selection from the health domains (Table 20) for nonspecific musculoskeletal spinal disorders, spinal cord injury and ankylosing spondylitis, these conditions having been taken as representative of the wide range of spinal disorders.

Specific causes

The various spinal diseases resulting from trauma are represented by spinal cord injury, there being a general recovery that progresses through stages of partial recovery with improved function but often static disease process. Acute spinal diseases resulting from mechanical factors are represented by a herniated nucleus pulposus, recovery progressing through a series of stages, with full recovery to normal health. The chronic spinal disease processes resulting from multiple factors are represented by ankylosing spondylitis, which progresses from normal health to potential severe disability.

The domains considered to be important in specific spinal diseases were as follows.

- Physical health: activities (activities of daily living, employment/work, leisure); impairment; mobility; pain and discomfort.
- Social health: activities; impairment.
- Mental health: emotional status; handicap/participation; social function.

The limitation of activities and the limitation of participation are the main primary outcomes and health indicators associated with spinal diseases. Data on these indicators may easily be collected in most countries through the adaptation of available self-reporting instruments.

Additional domains were proposed to include transportation, behaviour, the economic impact on individuals, the economic impact on society and the effect on families.

Nonspecific causes

Nonspecific musculoskeletal spinal disorders have a variable progression of recovery, including recovery to full health and deterioration to severe disability. The following domains were considered to be important in nonspecific spinal disorders.

- Physical health
  - activities;
    activities of living;
    employment/work;
    leisure;
  - impairment;
  - mobility;
  - pain and discomfort.
- Social health
  - activities;
  - impairment.
- Mental health
  - emotional status;
  - handicap/participation;
  - social function.

Pain, discomfort, limitation of activities and restriction of participation are the main primary outcomes and health indicators associated with nonspecific musculoskeletal spinal disorders. Data on these may easily be collected in most countries by adapting the available self-report instruments.

It was suggested that additional domains could be transportation, behaviour, the economic impact on the individual, the economic impact on society and the impact on families.

7.6.2 *Possible health states*

Hypothetical health states are shown for nonspecific spinal disorders, spinal cord injury and ankylosing spondylitis in Table 29. They provide representative examples of the heterogeneous and diverse disorders involving the spine. Table 30 simplifies complex disease processes that wax and wane: the rate of progression, the pace of deterioration and the degree of impairment in the different health domains at different disease stages are not uniform or synchronous.

Each chosen subdomain was assigned an anticipated performance rating on a scale that could be applied globally (i.e. a four-point scale in which 1 = "no impact", 2 = "mild impact", 3 = "moderate impact" and 4 = "severe impact"). This resulted in the sets of health states which form the columns of Table 29. No correlation was derived for disease stages.

7.6.3 *Suggested instruments for measuring selected health domains*

It was agreed that suitable instruments for recording the selected health domains include those shown in Table 30 (*180*). Some of these instruments depend on self-reporting and therefore require a certain degree of literacy. They also need to be translated into the language and revalidated to the culture of any country in which they are to be used.

7.7 Severe limb trauma

7.7.1 *Health domains*

Severe limb trauma often results in a significant impairment that can affect the ability to resume normal everyday living. For the young adult of working age, severe limb trauma often results in lost work days. Furthermore, a residual impairment may preclude returning to the job held before injury occurred. Also important to young people, especially if they were physically active before injury, is the effect on their participation in recreational and leisure activities. For older adults, severe limb trauma may preclude a return to independent living. At all ages, limb trauma is often associated with psychological

Table 29
Rating scale for health domains in various spinal disorders

Health Domain	Relevant Domains	Spinal disorder									
		Nonspecific spinal disorder				Spinal cord injury			Ankylosing spondylitis		
		Acute	Recurrent	Chronic	Chronic amplified	Acute	Subacute	Chronic	Acute	Subacute	Chronic
Overall well-being											
General health											
Physical health											
Activities/roles (activities of daily living)	X	2–4	1–4	2–4	3–4	4	2–4	3–4	1–2	2	3
Work (occupation)	X	1–4	1–4	1–4	3–4	4	2–4	1–4	1	1–2	2
Home											
Recreation (leisure)	X	1–4	1–4	1–4	2–4	4	3–4	1–4	1–2	2	2–3
Ambulation	X					4	3–4	2–4			
Eating	X					1–4	1–4	1–4			
Energy/vitality											
Mobility/fitness	X	2–4	1–4	1–4	3–4	4	3–4	2–4	2	3	3–4
Pain/discomfort (intensity)	X	2–4	2–4	2–4	2–4	2–4	2–4	1–4	2	2	1–2
Self-care											
Sleep/rest	X	1–3	1–2	1–3	2–4						

Social health (role)	X	1–4	1–4	1–4	1–4	4	3–4	1–3	1	1	1
Activities/roles	X		1–2	1–4	3–4	4	3–4	1–3			
Communication											
Interaction											
Support	X		1–2	1–3	2–4						
Mental health											
Activities/roles											
Alertness											
Anxiety/depression	X			1–4	3–4	4	2–4	1–2			
Cognition											
Emotional status	X	1–4	1–4	2–4	3–4	4	1–3	1–3	2	2	2
Outlook											
Self-esteem											
Handicap/participation (body impairment)	X	1–4	1–4	1–4	1–4	4	4	4	2	3	3
Environment											
Additional domains proposed											
Transportation	X	1–4	1–4	1–4	1–4	4	2–4	1–4	1	1	2–3
Behaviour	X	1–2	1–4	2–4	2–4	2–3	1–3	1–4	1	2	2
Economic impact on patient	X	1–2	1–4	2–4	3–4	4	2–4	1–4	1	1	2
Economic impact on society	X	1–2	1–2	1–3	3–4	4	2–4	1–4	2	2	2–4

X, applicable; 1, no impact; 2, mild impact; 3, moderate impact; 4, severe impact.

Table 30
Instruments for recording health domains for spinal disorders

Disease classification	Disease-specific	Generic
Spinal diseases	Oswestry	WHO Disability Assessment Schedule II (WHODAS II)
	Roland	Short Form Health Status Survey (SF-36)
	Kohlmann–Raspe	
	Brief Symptom Inventory	EuroQol (EQ-5D)
		Modified Health Assessment Questionnaire (HAQ)
		Activities of Daily Living (ADL)
		Visual Analog Pain Scale
		Quality of Well-Being Scale (QWB)
Nonspecific musculoskeletal spinal disorders	Oswestry	WHODAS II
	Roland	SF-36
	Kohlmann–Raspe	Chronic Pain Questionnaire
	Brief Symptom Inventory	Low Back Pain Nordic Questionnaire
		EuroQol (EQ-5D)
		Modified HAQ
		Spitzer Index
		ADL
		Visual Analog Pain Scale
		QWB

See Table 32 for full name and additional information on instruments.

consequences that interfere with everyday living and the overall quality of life. The impact of injury on post-traumatic stress and depression is of increasing importance in studies of recovery following major trauma (*132*). With regard to injuries that result in amputation, issues of body image and self-esteem are often of concern.

The following health domains were considered relevant for measuring the impact of upper and lower limb trauma (Table 31):

Table 31
Health-related domains and subdomains relevant to limb trauma

	Relevant domains	
	Upper limb	Lower limb
Overall well-being		
General health		
Perceived health	A	A
Change in health	A	A
Physical health		
Activities/roles		
Work	A	A
Home	A	A
Recreation	A/B	A/B
Ambulation	A	A
Eating	A	C
Energy/vitality	B	B
Mobility/fitness	C	A
Pain/discomfort	A	A
Self-care	A	A
Sleep/rest	B	B
Social health		
Activities/roles		
Communication	A (writing)	C
Interaction	B	B
Support		
Mental health		
Activities/roles		
Alertness	C	C
Anxiety/depression	A	A
Cognition	C	C
Emotional status	A	A
Outlook	A	A
Self-esteem	A	A
Handicap/participation		
Environment		
Additional domains proposed		
Fine motor	A	C
Movement — arms	A	C
Sexual function	B	A+
Driving	A	A

A, most important domain.

— self-care (especially among elderly people who sustain major traumas);
— symptoms (including bodily pain, numbness and stiffness);
— physical function (including ambulation/mobility, bending/lifting and stooping/crouching for lower limb trauma, and arm movement and hand and fine motor function for upper limb trauma);

- role functions (including those associated with work/school and home/family);
- social function (including social avoidance, recreational/leisure activities and intimate relations);
- mental health (including overall emotional well-being, anxiety/depression, post-traumatic stress and self-esteem/body image);
- general well-being (including energy/vitality and general health perceptions).

In order of decreasing importance, the domains and subdomains judged by the work group to be most relevant when measuring the overall impact of limb trauma are:

- work (or a return to independent living for older retired adults);
- recreation;
- ambulation/mobility for lower extremity trauma and hand/arm movement for upper limb trauma;
- pain;
- self-care;
- overall emotional well-being.

The course of recovery over these domains clearly depends on the type and severity of the injury, the age of the individual, any associated injuries and comorbidity, and other characteristics of the patient and the environment.

7.7.2 *Possible health states*

People suffering from severe limb trauma often proceed through several stages of recovery and adaptation to their residual limitations. The initial recovery from injury can take days, weeks or months, depending on the extent and nature of the injury. For the most severe injuries requiring extensive reconstruction, treatment and recovery can last considerably more than a year.

Once the initial treatment has been completed, a period of rehabilitation and reconditioning is often required in order to optimize recovery. However, even after extensive treatment and rehabilitation many persons are left with a residual impairment involving reduced strength, a limited range of motion or, in some cases, the loss of a limb. An adaptation to this impairment is often necessary through the use of special equipment and prosthetic and orthotic devices, or through a change in the physical environment (e.g. modifications to the person's home, workplace or vehicle). Long-term health states may involve the development of secondary medical conditions such as arthritis and osteomyelitis.

During the initial phase of recovery and rehabilitation the domains of physical function are key indicators of outcome, with special reference to ambulation for lower extremity trauma and to hand/arm movement for trauma of an upper extremity. As the wound heals, the emphasis on health outcomes quickly shifts to indicators of return to usual major activity and independent living. Indicators of long-term outcome will extend beyond the return to usual major activity and include emotional well-being, social interaction and general health.

When examining the consequences of limb trauma, it is important to adopt a framework that elucidates the relationships between different health states. The most direct way in which an injury affects the health of the individual involved is through the temporary and permanent impairments it causes. These impairments are typically assessed by means of standard metrics of a reduced range of motion, muscle strength and sensation. Impairments affect the individual through the functional limitations or activity limitations which they cause, including both physical limitations, e.g. in ambulation, lifting and bending and the manipulation of small objects, and psychological limitations, e.g. depression and anxiety.

Most important to patients, however, is the extent to which these limitations impact on their ability to participate fully in everyday life, including independent living, major role activity, recreation and social interaction. Although there is a strong correlation between the extent of injury and impairment, and between impairment and functional limitation or activity restriction, there is often no clear relationship between the severity of injury, the resulting impairment and restrictions on participation. This arises because some of the largest differentials in restriction on participation observed are related to numerous interacting personal, social and environmental factors that influence the overall course of recovery.

Although several studies have documented the important role that severity of illness, age and comorbidity play in determining the impact of injury, few have looked beyond this narrow set of predictors when developing appropriate models for explaining variations in impact. The few studies that have used a broader framework have documented how several characteristics of the individual and the environment are important in determining the trajectory of recovery. These include educational level, the amount and source of income, the availability of social support, motivation and health habits, including behaviour associated with alcohol consumption. With regard to vocational outcomes, the physical demands of the job held before injury occurred and the work setting, together with the type and amount of disability compensation, also influence the extent and rate of return to work.

For the purpose of identifying effective interventions that mediate the impact of injury on the quality of life, it is important to know how these multiple factors interact so as to influence the transitions between the different levels or complexities of function. Such knowledge is essential for an improved understanding of how and when to intervene.

7.7.3 *Suggested instruments for measuring selected health domains*

Several instruments, both generic and condition-specific, were reviewed for their applicability to the limb trauma population. Among the measures discussed were the following:

- — the Barthel Index for assessing limitations on activities of daily living (*181*);
- — the Functional Independence Measure (FIM) for assessing limitations on instrumental activities of daily living (*182*);
- — the SIP (*183*);
- — the SF-36 and SF-12 health surveys (*184*, *185*);
- — the Child Health Questionnaire (CHQ) (*186*);
- — the QWB (*187*);
- — the Health Utilities Index (HUI) (*188*);
- — EuroQol (*189*);
- — the Functional Capacity Index (FCI) (*190*);
- — the Musculoskeletal Function Assessment (MFA) and the Shortened Musculoskeletal Function Assessment (SMFA) (*191*).

The first eight measures are generic measures of functional status. The FCI is specific to trauma, and the MFA and SMFA were developed for assessing the impact of musculoskeletal conditions, including injury. The Barthel Index, FIM, SIP, SF-36, CHQ and MFA are psychometric measures or health status profiles that describe the health status of a person across a comprehensive set of domains, yielding separate scores for each domain together with one or more summary scores providing an overall measure of physical versus mental or psychosocial health.

The QWB, FCI, EuroQol and HUI are preference-based measures providing a single summary score, typically ranging from 0 (representing death) to 1 (optimal health). These scores reflect the preferences of patients or consumers for different health profiles and are derived on the basis of decision theory and economic principles. Unlike health profiles, preference-based measures combine death and quality of life into a single metric and can be used together with survival data in calculating QALYs.

In reviewing these measures the workgroup made the following observations.

- No single measure seemed to capture all the dimensions outlined above with sufficient depth to fully characterize the impact of limb trauma. At the same time the participants agreed that, for the purpose of broad, population-based monitoring, it was important to choose brief, practical measures that could be translated across many different cultures.
- Although the QWB, HUI, FCI and EuroQol were attractive because they could be used to derive QALY-like measures of the burden of injury, the use of measures combining states and values into one number presented a difficulty in that the value placed on various health states could differ substantially between cultures.
- Although the FIM was widely advocated as a measure of injury outcome, like other measures of activities of daily living and instrumental activities of daily living it was not sensitive to variation in outcome at the higher end of functioning that would be more typical of many limb injuries. In addition, the FIM did not incorporate broader issues of disability and quality of life, such as role activity, psychological well-being and general health perceptions.
- Although some controversy still existed about the relative benefits of generic versus condition-specific or disease-specific measures, most members of the work group agreed that the use of a generic measure was important as it facilitated a comparison across different conditions and injuries, populations, investigations and interventions. Generic measures were particularly useful when the outcome of multiple traumas was being measured, since multiple body systems were involved and there were consequences affecting various aspects of function. However, the generic measures might not be sensitive to many of the specific limitations resulting from limb injuries, especially moderately severe injuries of the hand and upper extremities.
- There was a lack of measures specific to children, although the recent development of the CHQ provided a promising generic measure that might be well suited to studying the consequences of limb injury in this age group.
- It was vitally important to collect data based on uniform measures of functional status/quality of life so that a start could be made on deriving consistent estimates of the impact of limb trauma across countries. A preliminary assessment was that the use of the MFA (or possibly the SMFA), together with a short generic measure such

as the SF-36 or SF-12 (for adults) and the CHQ (for children), would provide a reasonably sound indication of the impact of limb trauma. These instruments are described in more detail in Section 8.

8. Inventory of published assessment instruments for musculoskeletal conditions

8.1 Introduction

The purpose of this inventory is to serve as a resource for use during the Bone and Joint Decade Monitor Project when information or questions arise about instruments or measures of musculoskeletal health.

8.2 Data collected

A standard set of data was collected for each instrument or measure. In order to create a database of manageable size, only a small core data set was included. The data collection form covered various aspects of the instruments including scope, reliability/validity, areas assessed and language availability (the form can be found at http://www.aaos.org/wordhtml/research/bjdecad/list01.htm).

8.2.1 *Instrument name*

The formal title of each instrument is included (e.g. the Nottingham Health Profile), or an assigned title is given (e.g. the Disability Assessment Measure) if there was no formal title.

8.2.2 *Bibliographic citation*

The citation(s) that include each instrument, its characteristics, its reliability and its validity are listed. If it was not possible to obtain the primary reference, a secondary source was used. In some instances two citations were given because all the relevant information was not included in one.

8.2.3 *Instruments designed for or used with various populations*

Most instruments are designed for use with either children or adults, the population in question being noted on the instrument inventory form. When an instrument is applicable to both children and adults, or where versions are available for both populations, this is indicated. In cases in which an instrument was designed for adolescents, the instrument is listed under children.

Instruments that were designed for and/or used with the general population are designated as general population surveys. Instruments designed for or applicable to a specific population are listed as applicable for clinical trials.

8.2.4 *Disease conditions*

An indication is given as to whether the instruments identified have been used with the major categories of musculoskeletal conditions being addressed in the Bone and Joint Decade Monitor Project. One or more conditions may be ticked, as applicable.

8.2.5 *Reliability data*

The inventory is primarily limited to instruments for which some reliability data were available. Exceptions are made in the case of long-standing instruments that would be familiar to many physicians caring for people with musculoskeletal conditions. No evaluation was made as to whether the reliability data fell within acceptable psychometric standards. For the purposes of the database the major types relate to internal consistency and test/retest reliability measures.

8.2.6 *Validity data*

The inventory is primarily limited to instruments for which some validity data are available, although exceptions were made in the case of long-standing instruments that would be familiar to many physicians caring for individuals with musculoskeletal disease. No evaluation was made as to whether the validity data lay within acceptable psychometric standards.

For the purposes of the database the major types relate to content, construct, concurrent, criterion and predictive validity. Authors differ in their classification of certain types of validity. Some, for example, ascribe data to a criterion validity category, whereas others state that there is no gold standard and place the same type of data in a construct validity category. The inventory uses each author's classification. A classification was assigned where no classification was indicated.

8.2.7 *Type of indicator*

Health indicators were placed in either a generic category or a specific category. The generic category includes health status measures and utility measures. Health status measures are multidimensional and are generally concerned with physical, emotional and social functioning. Specific measures are designed for a specific disease or condition or for a specific population. Economic indicators refer to ways of measuring the economic impact on society.

8.2.8 *Areas measured*

Instruments may focus on different areas. Most measure either the disability resulting from a disease or injury, or the overall health-related quality of life, which generally includes physical, emotional and social functioning.

Few instances were found of instruments that measure resource utilization. Cost measures are rarely included in instruments, although some of the utility measures can be used in determining cost.

8.2.9 *Administration*

Some instruments are categorized as self-reported or, in the case of young children, reported by parents. Others require an interviewer or observer to complete them. One of the advantages of self-report instruments is that they are less costly to administer.

8.2.10 *Time to complete*

As a measure of response burden, the reported time to complete an instrument, when available, is recorded.

8.2.11 *Language*

The search for instruments was limited to the English language, so almost all those in the database are available in English. Minor exceptions occurred when an instrument designed in another language was reported in an English-language journal. Many instruments have been translated into languages other than English, and the major languages are listed.

8.2.12 *Copy available*

A copy was requested of each instrument that seemed to be comparatively widely used. A filled-in box indicates that a printed copy was available for reference.

8.3 Search methodology

Several sources were used to obtain the list of instruments.

8.3.1 *Experts in musculoskeletal conditions*

A series of experts, including both individuals and government agencies, were asked to give suggestions for actual instruments or for sources that reviewed instruments.

8.3.2 *Existing databases*

Several existing computerized databases were reviewed. The Health and Psychosocial Instruments database seemed to be best suited as a resource for the purposes of locating health and economic instruments. It covered publications from 1985 onwards.

Multiple searches were conducted by:

— the titles of the instruments, when known;
— the author(s) of the instruments;
— keywords such as "quality of life", "activities of daily living", "life satisfaction" and "utility measure".

8.3.3 *Review text*

The second edition of *Quality of life and pharmacoeconomics in clinical trials* (*192*) was reviewed by the Scientific Group for instruments. The reference lists of relevant chapters were reviewed, and they provided additional candidates for inclusion.

The search strategy was not designed to be exhaustive but to identify instruments that would be known to and/or used by the musculoskeletal care provider community.

8.4 Selected instrument listings

A list of all the identified instruments and primary citations is given in Table 32. A database of this information and all additionally collected data on these instruments is available at http://www.aaos.org/wordhtml/research/bjdecad/list01.htm. Instruments contained in the database can be listed alphabetically or by the following categories:

— Instruments for assessing adults
— Instruments for assessing children
— Cost measure instruments
— Disability instruments
— Economic instruments
— General musculoskeletal conditions
— Generic health profile instruments
— Generic utility measures
— Limb trauma instruments
— Osteoarthritis instruments
— Osteoporosis instruments
— Quality-of-life instruments
— Resource utilization instruments
— Rheumatoid arthritis instruments
— Specific instruments
— Spine disorders instruments.

Table 32
Reference information for instruments assessing musculoskeletal conditions

Instrument	Citations[a]
12-Item Short-Form Health Survey (SF-12)	**Ware JE, Kosinski M, Keller SD.** A 12-item short-form health survey. *Medical care*, 1996, **34**:220–233.
AAOS Disabilities of the Arm, Shoulder and Hand (DASH)	**Hudak P, Amadio PC, Bombardier C and the Upper Extremity Collaborative Group.** Development of an upper extremity outcome measure: the DASH (Disabilities of the Arm, Shoulder and Hand). *American journal of industrial medicine*, 1996, **29**:602–608.
	Marx R. *A comparison of clinimetric and psychometric techniques for item reduction in the development of an upper extremity disability measure* [Master's thesis]. Toronto, University of Toronto Press, 1996.
	Upper Extremity Collaborative Group. Measuring disability and symptoms of the upper limb: a validation study of the DASH Questionnaire. *Arthritis and rheumatism*, 1996, **39**:S112.
AAOS Lower Limb Questionnaire	**Daltroy L et al.** AAOS lower limb outcomes scales: reliability, validity, and sensitivity to change. (Submitted for publication).
AAOS Short Form Musculoskeletal Assessment (SFMA)	**Martin DP et al.** Comparison of the Musculoskeletal Function Assessment Questionnaire with the Short Form-36, the Western Ontario and McMaster Universities Osteoarthritis Index, and the Sickness Impact Profile health-status measures. *Journal of bone and joint surgery*, 1997, **79**:1323–1335.
AAOS Spine Questionnaire	**Daltroy LH et al.** The North American Spine Society Lumbar Spine Outcome Assessment Instrument. Reliability and validity tests. *Spine*, 1996, **21**:741–749.
	Daltroy LH et al. Lumbar and Cervical Spine Questionnaire. Reliability and validity tests. Work in progress.
AAOS/POSNA Pediatric Questionnaire	**Daltroy LH et al.** The POSNA Pediatric Musculoskeletal Functional Health Questionnaire: report on reliability, validity, and sensitivity to change. *Journal of pediatric orthopaedics*, 1998, **18**:561–571.
ACL Injuries	**Pynsent PB, Fairbank JCT, Carr A.** *Outcome measures in orthopedics.* Oxford: Butterworth-Heinemann, 1993.
ACR Preliminary Core Set of Disease Activity Measures for Rheumatoid Arthritis	**Felson DT et al.** The American College of Rheumatology preliminary core set of disease activity measures for rheumatoid arthritis clinical trials. *Arthritis and rheumatism*, 1993, **36**:729–740.
Activities of Daily Living (ADL) Scale	**Katz S et al.** Studies of illness in the aged. The Index of ADL: a standardized measure of biological and psychosocial function. *Journal of the American Medical Association*, 1963, **185**:914–919.
Activities of Daily Living Scale — "Adapted"	**Hedrick SC et al.** Adult day health care evaluation study: methodology and implementation. *Health services research*, **25**:936.

Table 32 (*Continued*)

Instrument	Citations[a]
Activities of Daily Living Scale — "Modified" — "Selected Items"	**Gill TM, Williams CS, Tinetti ME.** Assessing risk for the onset of functional dependence among older adults: the role of physical performance. *Journal of the American Geriatrics Society*, 1995, **43**:603–609.
Activities of Daily Living Scale — Japanese	**Nagatomo I et al.** A study of the quality of life of elderly people using psychological testing. *International journal of geriatric psychiatry*, 1997, **12**:599–608.
Aggregate Functional Performance Time Measure (AFPT)	**Hurley MV et al.** Sensorimotor changes and functional performance in patients with knee osteoarthritis. *Annals of the rheumatic diseases*, 1997, **56**:641–648.
Ankle Clinical Rating System	**Kitaoka HB et al.** Clinical Rating System for the ankle-hindfoot, midfoot, hallux, and lesser toes. *Foot and ankle international*, 1994, **15**:349–353.
Ankylosing Spondylitis Questionnaire	**Kraag G et al.** The effects of comprehensive home physiotherapy and supervision on patients with ankylosing spondylitis: a randomized controlled trial. *Journal of rheumatology*, 1990, **17**:228–233.
Arthritis Impact Measurement Scales (AIMS)	**Meenan RF, Gertman PM, Mason JH.** Measuring health status in arthritis: the Arthritis Impact Measurement Scale. *Arthritis and rheumatism*, 1980, **23**:146–152.
Arthritis Impact Measurement Scales-2 (AIMS-2)	**Meenan RF et al.** AIMS2: the content and properties of a revised and expanded arthritis impact measurement scales health status questionnaire. *Arthritis and rheumatism*, 1992, **35**:1–10.
	Potts MK, Brandt KD. Evidence of the validity of the arthritis impact measurement scales. *Arthritis and rheumatism*, 1987, **30**:93–96.
Arthritis Impact Measurement Scales-2 — Short Form	**Guillemin F et al.** The AIMS2-SF: a short form of the Arthritis Impact Measurement Scales-2. French Quality of Life in Rheumatology Group. *Arthritis and rheumatism*, 1997, **40**:1267–1274.
Arthritis Self-Efficacy Scale	**Lorig K et al.** Development and evaluation of a scale to measure perceived self-efficacy in people with arthritis. *Arthritis and rheumatism*, 1989, **32**:37–44.
AUSCAN Hand Osteoarthritis Index	**Bellamy N et al.** Development of a disease specific health status measure for hand osteoarthritis clinical trials. Assessment of reliability and validity. *Journal of rheumatology*, 1997, **24**:1425.
	Bellamy N et al. Development of the Australian/Canadian (AUSCAN) osteoarthritis (OA) hand index. *Arthritis and rheumatism*, 1997, **40**:S110.
Barthel Index	**Mahoney FI, Barthel DW.** Functional evaluation: the Barthel Index. *Maryland State medical journal*, 1965, **14**:61–65.
Carpal Tunnel Syndrome Symptom Severity Scale	**Levine DW et al.** A self-administered questionnaire for the assessment of severity of symptoms and functional status in carpal tunnel syndrome. *Journal of bone and joint surgery*, 1993, **75**:1585–1592.

Table 32 (*Continued*)

Instrument	Citations[a]
Carpal Tunnel Syndrome Functional Status Scale	**Levine DW et al.** A self-administered questionnaire for the assessment of severity of symptoms and functional status in carpal tunnel syndrome. *Journal of bone and joint surgery*, 1993, **75**:1585–1592.
Charnley Method for Hip Evaluation	**Charnley J.** The long-term results of low-friction arthroplasty of the hip performed as a primary intervention. *Journal of bone and joint surgery*, 1972, **54**: 61–76.
Child Activities of Daily Living Scale (CADL)	**Varni JW et al.** Chronic musculoskeletal pain and functional status in juvenile rheumatoid arthritis: an empirical model. *Pain*, 1988, **32**:1–7.
Child Health and Illness Profile — Adolescent Edition	**Starfield B et al.** The Adolescent Child Health and Illness Profile. *Medical care*, 1995, **33**:553–566.
Child Health Questionnaire (CHQ)	**Landgraf JM et al.** Canadian-French, German and UK versions of the Child Health Questionnaire. *Quality of life research*, 1998, **7**:433–445.
Childhood Health Assessment Questionnaire (CHAQ)	**Singh G et al.** Measurement of health status in children with juvenile rheumatoid arthritis. *Arthritis and rheumatism*, 1994, **37**:1761–1769.
	Billings AG et al. Psychosocial adaptation in juvenile rheumatic disease: a controlled evaluation. *Health psychology*, 1987, **6**:343–359.
Convery Polyarticular Disability Index	**Convery FR et al.** Polyarticular disability: a functional assessment. *Archives of physical and medical rehabilitation*, 1997, **58**:494–499.
Criterion-Referenced Measure of Goal Attainment Tool	**King IM.** Measuring health goal attainment in patients. In: Waltz CF and Strickland OL, eds. *Measurement of nursing outcomes: measuring client outcomes*, Vol. 1, New York, NY, Springer, 1988, 108–127.
Dartmouth COOP Charts	**Nelson EC, Wasson JH, Kirk JW.** Assessment of function in routine clinical practice: description of the COOP Chart Method and preliminary findings. *Journal of chronic disease*, 1987, **40**:555–635.
	Nelson FC et al. The functional status of patients: how can it be measured in physician's offices? *Medical care*, 1990, **28**:1111–1126.
Disabilities of the Arm, Shoulder and Hand (DASH) Outcome Measure	**Hudak PL et al.** Development of an upper extremity outcome measure: The DASH (disabilities of the arm, shoulder and head). *American journal of industrial medicine*, 1996, **29**:602–608.
	Hudak PL et al. Erratum: [Development of an upper extremity outcome measure: The DASH (Disabilities of the Arm, Shoulder and Hand). American Journal of Industrial Medicine, 1996; 29:602–608]. *American journal of industrial medicine*, 1996, **30**:602–608.
Disease Activity	**Zurier RB et al.** Gamma-linolenic acid treatment of rheumatoid arthritis: a randomized placebo-controlled trial. *Arthritis and rheumatism*. 1996, **39**:1808–1817.

Table 32 (*Continued*)

Instrument	Citations[a]
Disease Repercussion Profile (DRP)	**Carr AJ.** A patient-centred approach to evaluation and treatment in rheumatoid arthritis: the development of a clinical tool to measure patient-perceived handicap. *British journal of rheumatology*, 1996, **35**:921–932.
Duke Health Profile (DUKE)	**Parkerson GR Jr, Broadhead WE, Tse CK.** The Duke Health Profile: a 17-item measure of health and dysfunction. *Medical care*, 1990, **28**:1056–1072.
Duke-UNC Health Profile (DUHP)	**Parkerson GR Jr et al.** The Duke-UNC Health Profile: an adult health status instrument for primary care. *Medical care*, 1981, **19**:806–828.
Economic Evaluation of Health Care Programmes	**Drummond MF, Stoddart GL, Torrance GW.** *Methods for economic evaluation of health care programmes.* Oxford, Oxford Medical Publications, 1986.
EuroQol Instrument (EQ-5D)	**EuroQol Group.** EuroQol — a new facility for the measurement of health-related quality of life. *Health policy*, 1990, **16**:199–208.
	Hurst NP et al. Measuring health-related quality of life in rheumatoid arthritis: validity responsiveness and reliability of EuroQol (EQ-5D). *British journal of rheumatology*, 1997, **36**:551–559.
	Johnson JA, Pickard AS. Comparison of the EQ-5D and SF-12 health surveys in a general population survey in Alberta, Canada. *Medical care*, 1999, **38**:115–121.
Foot Function Index	**Budiman-Mak E, Conrad KJ, Roach KE.** The foot function index: a measure of foot pain and disability. *Clinical epidemiology*, 1991, **44**:561–570.
Functional Capacity Index (FCI)	**MacKenzie EJ et al.** The development of the functional capacity index. *Journal of trauma-injury, infection and critical care*, 1996, **41**:799–807.
Functional Disability Inventory — Child Version (FDI-Child)	**Walker LS, Green JW.** The Functional Disability Inventory: measuring a neglected dimension of child health status. *Journal of pediatric psychology*, 1991, **16**:39–58.
Functional Independence Measure (FIM)	**Granger CV, Hamilton BB.** *Functional Independence Measure (FIM).* Buffalo, NY, State University of New York at Buffalo, 1987.
	Stineman MG et al. The Functional Independence Measure: tests of scaling assumptions, structure, and reliability across 200 diverse impairment categories. *Archives of physical and medical rehabilitation*, 1996, **77**:1101–1108.
Functional Independence Measure — "Modified"	**Saxton J et al.** Maintenance of mobility in residents of an Alzheimer special care facility. *International psychogeriatrics*, 1998, **10**:213–224.
Functional Independence Measure for Children (WeeFIM)	**Granger CV, Hamilton BB, Kayton R.** *Guide for the use of the Functional Independence Measure for Children (WeeFIM).* New York, NY, Research Foundation, State University of New York, 1989.
	Msall ME et al. The Functional Independence Measure for Children (WeeFIM). *Clinical pediatrics*, 1994, **33**:421–430.

Table 32 (*Continued*)

Instrument	Citations[a]
Functional Status Index	**Jette AM.** Functional Status Index: reliability of a chronic disease evaluation instrument. *Archives of physical and medical rehabilitation*, 1980, **61**:395–401.
	Ganiats TG, Palinkas LAS, Kaplan RM. Comparison of Quality of Well-Being Scale and Functional Status Index in patients with atrial fibrillation. *Medical care*, 1992, **30**:958–964.
	Jette AM. The Functional Status Index: reliability and validity of a self-report functional disability measure. *Journal of rheumatology*, 1987, **14**:15.
Functional Status Questionnaire (FSQ)	**Jette AM, Davies AR, Cleary PD et al.** The Functional Status Questionnaire: reliability and validity when used in primary care. *Journal of general internal medicine*, 1986, **1**:143–149.
Functional Status Questionnaire — General (for Children)	**Lewis CC, Pantell RH, Kieckhofer GM.** Assessment of children's health status: field test of new approaches. *Medical care*, 1989, **27** (suppl. 3):54–65.
General Life Satisfaction Measure	**Mehta S.** Relationship between acculturation and mental health for Asian Indian immigrants in the United States. *Genetic, social and general psychology monographs*, 1998, **127**:61–78.
General Quality of Life Inventory — Chinese	**Li L, Young D.** The development of the General Quality of Life Inventory. *China mental health journal*, 1995, **9**:227–231.
General Well-Being Schedule	**Dupuy DF.** Utility of the National Center for Health Statistics' General Well-Being in the assessment of self-representations of subjective well-being and distress. Paper presented at the National Conference on the Evaluation of Drug Alcohol and Mental Health Programs, 1975.
	Dupuy HR. *A concurrent validational study of the NCHS General Well-Being Schedule*. Hyattsville, MD, National Center for Health Statistics, US Department of Health, Education and Welfare, 1977 (DHEW Publication No. HRA 78-1347).
GERI-AIMS (Arthritis Impact Measurement Scales)	**Hughes SL et al.** The GERI-AIMS. Reliability and validity of the Arthritis Impact Measurement Scales adapted for elderly respondents. *Arthritis and rheumatism*, 1991, **34**:856–865.
Goteborg Quality of Life Instrument — Well-Being Scale — Swedish	**Tibblin G et al.** The Goteborg Quality of Life Instrument — an assessment of well-being and symptoms among men born 1913 and 1923. *Scandinavian journal of primary health care supplement*, 1990, **1** (suppl.):33–38.
Groningen Activity Restriction Scale	**Kempen GI, Suurmeijer JP.** The development of a hierarchical polychotomous ADL-IADL scale for noninstitutional elders. *Gerontologist*, 1990, **30**:497–502.
	Surrmeijer TP et al. The Groningen Activity Restriction Scale for measuring disability: its utility in international comparisons. *American journal of public health*, 1994, **84**:1270–1273.

Table 32 (*Continued*)

Instrument	Citations[a]
Gross Motor Function Measure	**Russell DJ et al.** The gross motor function measure: a means to evaluate the effects of physical therapy. *Developmental medicine and child neurology*, 1989, **31**:341–352.
Hannover Activities of Daily Living Questionnaire	**Kohlmann T, Raspe HH.** Die patientennahe Diagnostik von Funktionseinschräankungen im Alltag. [A patient-centred assessment of functional impairment in daily living.] *Psychomedizin* [Psychological medecine], 1994, **6**:21–27.
Harris Hip Scale	**Harris WH.** Traumatic arthritis of the hip after dislocation and acetabular fractures: treatment by mold arthroplasty. *Journal of bone and joint surgery*, 1969, **51**:737–755.
Health Assessment Questionnaire (HAQ) for Arthritis	**Fries JC et al.** Measurement of patient outcome in arthritis. *Arthritis and rheumatism*, 1980, **23**:137–145.
	Ramey DR, Fries JF, Singh G. The Health Assessment Questionnaire 1995 — status and review. In: Spilker B, ed. *Quality of life and pharmacoeconomics, 2nd ed.* Philadelphia, PA, Lippincott-Raven, 1996:227–237.
Health Assessment Questionnaire for Spondyloarthropathies (HAQ-S)	**Daltroy LH et al.** A modification of the Health Assessment Questionnaire of the Spondyloarthropathies. *Journal of rheumatology*, 1990, **17**:946–950.
	Gudex C, Kind P. *The HMQ: measuring health status in the community.* Discussion Paper No. 93. York, University of York, Centre for Health Economics, 1991.
Health Measurement Questionnaire Health Utilities Index (HUI)	**Feeny D et al.** Multi-attribute health status classification systems: Health Utilities Index. *Pharmacoeconomics*, 1995, **7**:490–502.
	Torrance GW et al. Multi-attribute preference functions: Health Utilities Index. *Pharmacoeconomics*, 1995, **7**:503–520.
Health-Related Quality-of-Life Rating Task	**Hadorn DC, Hays RD.** Multimethod analysis of health-related quality-of-life measures. *Medical care*, 1991, **29**:829–840.
Hip Function (Ilstrup and Nolan)	**Ilstrup DM et al.** Factors influencing the results in 2,012 total hip arthroplasties. *Clinical orthopaedics & related research*, 1973, **95**:250–262.
Hip Function (Larson Rating Scale)	**Larson CB.** Rating scale for hip disabilities. *Clinical orthopedics*, 1963, **31**:85–93
Hip Function (Merle d'Aubigne and Postal)	**Merle d'Aubigne R, Postal M.** Functional results of hip arthroplasty with acrylic prosthesis. *Journal of bone and joint surgery*, 1954, **36**:451–475.
Hip Rating System — Hospital for Special Surgery	**Salvati EA, Wilson PD Jr.** Long-term results of femoral-head replacement. *Journal of bone and joint surgery*, 1973, **55**:516–524.
Hip Replacement, Total — Terminology	**Johnston RC et al.** Clinical and radiographic evaluation of total hip replacement: a standard system of terminology for reporting results. *Journal of bone and joint surgery*, 1990, **72**:161–168.

Table 32 (*Continued*)

Instrument	Citations[a]
Index of Severity for Knee Disease — French (ISK)	**Lequesne MG et al.** Indexes of severity for osteoarthritis of the hip and knee. Validation — value in comparison with other assessment tests. *Scandinavian journal of rheumatology supplement*, 1987, **65**:85–89.
Instrumental Activities of Daily Living — Male, Female	**Lawton HP, Brody EM.** Assessment of older people: self-maintaining and instrumental activities of daily living. *Gerontologist*, 1969, **9**:179–186.
Instrumental Activities of Daily Living — Older Adults	**Lawton HP, Brody EM.** Assessment of older people: self-maintaining and instrumental activities of daily living. *Gerontologist*, 1969, **9**:179–186.
International Knee Documentation Committee (IKDC)	**Hefti F et al.** Evaluation of knee ligament injuries with the IKDC form. *Knee surgery, sports traumatology, arthroscopy*, 1993, **1**:226–234.
Jebsen Hand Function	**Jebsen RH et al.** An objective and standardized test of hand function. *Archives of physical medicine and rehabilitation*, 1969, **50**:311–319.
Juvenile Arthritis Functional Assessment Report (JAFAR-C, JAFAR-P)	**Howe S et al.** Development of a disability measurement tool for juvenile rheumatoid arthritis. *Arthritis and rheumatism*, 1991, **34**:873–880.
Juvenile Arthritis Functional Assessment Scale (JAFAS)	**Lovell DH et al.** Development of a disability measurement tool for juvenile rheumatoid arthritis. *Arthritis and rheumatism*, 1989, **32**:1390–1395.
Juvenile Arthritis Self-Report Index (JASI)	**Wright FV et al.** A functional status index for juvenile arthritis (JA). *Physiotherapy Canada*, 1992, **44** (conference proceedings insert):6.
Keitel Function Test	**Kalla A et al.** Clinical assessment of disease activity in rheumatoid arthritis. Evaluation of a functional test. *Annals of the rheumatic diseases*, 1988, **47**:773–779.
Klein-Bell ADL Scale	**Klein RM, Bell B.** *The Klein-Bell ADL scale manual.* Seattle, WA, University of Washington Medical School, Health Sciences Resource Center, 1979. **Klein RM, Bell B.** Self-care skills: behavioral measurement with the Klein-Bell ADL Scale. *Archives of physical medicine and rehabilitation*, 1982, **63**:335–338.
Knee Assessment — ACL	**Mohtadi NG.** Quality of life assessment as an outcome in anterior cruciate ligament reconstructive surgery. In: Jackson DW et al., eds. *The anterior cruciate ligament current and future concepts.* New York, NY, Raven Press, 1993:439–444.
Knee Injury and Osteoarthritis Outcome Score (KOOS)	**Roos EM et al.** Knee Injury and Osteoarthritis Outcome Score (KOOS) — development of a self-administered outcome measure. *Journal of orthopaedic sports physical therapy*, 1998, **78**:88–96.
Kohlmann-Raspe Instrument for the Spine	**Kohlmann T, Raspe HH.** Hannover Functional Questionnaire in ambulatory diagnosis of functional disability caused by backache. *Rehabilitation* (*Stuttg*), 1996, **35**:I–VIII.
Knee Society Clinical Rating System	**Insall JN et al.** Rationale of the Knee Society clinical rating system. *Clinical orthopaedics & related research*, 1989, **248**:13–14.

Table 32 (*Continued*)

Instrument	Citations[a]
Lee Functional Index in Rheumatoid Arthritis	**Lee P et al.** Evaluation of a functional index in rheumatoid arthritis. *Scandinavian journal of rheumatology*, 1973, **2**:71–77.
Life Satisfaction Index A, B	**Neugarten BL, Havighurst RJ, Tobin SS.** The measurement of life satisfaction. *Journal of gerontology*, 1961, **16**:134–143. **Adams DL.** Analysis of a life satisfaction index. *Journal of gerontology*, 1969, **24**:470–474. **Fuhrer MJ et al.** Relationship of life satisfaction to impairment, disability and handicap among persons with spinal cord injury living in the community. *Archives of physical medicine and rehabilitation*, 1992, **73**:552–557.
Life Satisfaction Index Z	**Adams DL.** Analysis of a life satisfaction index. *Journal of gerontology*, 1969, **24**:470–474.
McMaster Health Index Questionnaire (MHIQ)	**Chambers LW et al.** The McMaster Health Index questionnaire as a measure of quality of life for patients with rheumatoid arthritis. *Journal of rheumatology*, 1982, **9**:780–784.
MACTAR Patient Preference Disability Questionnaire (MACTAR)	**Tugwell P et al.** The MACTAR Patient Preference Disability Questionnaire, an individual functional priority approach for assessing improvement in physical disability in clinical trials in rheumatoid arthritis. *Journal of rheumatology*, 1987, **14**:446–451.
Mayo Clinic Forefoot Scoring System	**Kitaoka KA, Holiday AD.** Metatarsal head resection for bunionette: long-term follow-up. *Foot and ankle*, 1991, **11**:345–349. **Pochatko DJ et al.** Distal chevron osteotomy with lateral release for treatment of hallux valgus deformity. *Foot and ankle*, 1994, **15**:457–461.
Michigan Hand Outcomes Questionnaire	**Chung KC et al.** Reliability and validity testing of the Michigan Hand Outcomes Questionnaire. *Journal of hand surgery*, 1998, **23**:575–587.
Mini-Duke-UNC Health Profile	**Blake RL, Vandiver TA.** The reliability and validity of a ten-item measure of functional status. *Journal of family practice*, 1986, **23**:455–459.
Modified Health Assessment Questionnaire (MHAQ)	**Pincus T et al.** Assessment of patient satisfaction in activities of daily living using a Modified Stanford Health Assessment Questionnaire. *Arthritis and rheumatism*, 1983, **26**:1346–1353.
Musculoskeletal Function Assessment Instrument	**Martin DP et al.** Development of a musculoskeletal function assessment instrument. *Journal of orthopaedic research*, 1996, **14**:173–181. **Engelberg R et al.** Musculoskeletal function assessment instrument: criterion and construct validity. *Journal of orthopaedic research*, 1996, **14**:182–192.
National Health Interview Survey — 1995 — Selected Items	**National Center for Health Statistics.** *National Health Interview Survey*. Hyattsville, MD, National Center for Health Statistics, 1984.

Table 32 (*Continued*)

Instrument	Citations[a]
Nottingham Health Profile (NHP)	**Hunt SM, McEwen J, McKanna SP.** *Measuring health status.* London, Croom Helm, 1986.
Noyes Knee Rating System	**Noyes FR ed.** *The Noyes Knee Rating System,* 2nd ed. Cincinnati, OH, Cincinnati Sports Medicine Research and Education Foundation, 1995.
Osteoporosis Assessment Questionnaire (OPAQ)	**Randell AG et al.** Quality of life in osteoporosis: reliability, consistency, and validity of the osteoporosis assessment questionnaire. *Journal of rheumatology*, 1998, **25**:1171–1179.
Oswestry Low Back Pain Disability Questionnaire	**Fairbank JCT et al.** The Oswestry Low Back Pain Disability Questionnaire. *Physiotherapy*, 1980, **66**:271–273. **Baker D et al.** The Oswestry Disability Index revisited: its reliability, repeatability, and validity and a comparison with St Thomas' Disability Index. In: Roland M, Jenner JR, eds. *Back pain: new approaches to rehabilitation.* Manchester, Manchester University Press, 1989:174–184.
Patient-Generated Index (PGI)	**Ruta DA et al.** A new approach to the measurement of quality of life: the Patient-Generated Index. *Medical care*, 1994, **32**:1109–1126.
Patient-Specific Index (PSI) — Hip Rating Scale	**Wright J, Rudicel S, Feinstein A.** Ask patients what they want. *Journal of bone and joint surgery*, 1994, **76**:229–234.
Pediatric Evaluation of Disability Inventory (PEDI)	**Haley SW et al.** *Pediatric Evaluation of Disability Inventory (PEDI). Development, standardization and administration manual.* Boston, MA, New England Medical Center Hospital, 1992.
Perceived Health Status	**Engel NS.** On the vicissitudes of health appraisal. *Advances in nursing care*, 1984, **7**:12–23.
Perceived Health Status Measure — IADL Functional Status Measures	**Myers AM.** The clinical Swiss army knife: empirical evidence on the validity of IADL functional status measures. *Medical care*, 1992, **30** (suppl. 5):MS96–111.
Pfeffer Functional Activity Questionnaire — Older Adults	**Pfeffer RI et al.** Measurement of functional activities of older adults in the community. *Journal of gerontology*, 1982, **37**:323–329.
Physical Health Measure	**Belloc NB, Breslow N, Hochstin J.** Measurement of physical health in a general population survey. *American journal of epidemiology*, 1971, **93**:328–336.
Psychological General Well-Being Index (PG WB)	**Dupuy HJ.** The Psychological General Well-Being (PG WB) Index. In: Wenger NK et al., eds. *Assessment of quality of life in clinical trials of cardiovascular therapies.* New York, NY, Le Jacq Publishing, 1984:170–183.
PULSES Profile	**Moskowitz E, McCann CB.** Classification of disability in the chronically ill and ageing. *Journal of chronic disease*, 1957, **5**:342–346.
Quality of Life Enjoyment and Satisfaction (Q-LES-Q)	**Endicott J et al.** Quality of Life Enjoyment and Satisfaction Questionnaire: a new measure. *Psychopharmacology bulletin*, 1993, **29**:321–326.

Table 32 (*Continued*)

Instrument	Citations[a]
Quality of Life Index (QL-Index)	**Spitzer WO et al.** Measuring the quality of life of cancer patients. A concise QL-Index for use by physicians. *Journal of chronic disease*, 1981, **34**:585–597.
Quality of Life Questionnaire	**Evans DR, Cope WE.** *Quality of Life Questionnaire (QLQ).* North Tonawanda, NY, Multi-Health Systems, 1989.
Quality-of-Life Questionnaire (2)	**Grimm HR Jr et al.** Relationships of quality-of-life measures to long-term lifestyle and drug treatment in the treatment of mild hypertension study. *Archives of internal medicine*, 1997, **157**:638–648.
Quality of Life Questionnaire of the European Foundation for Osteoporosis (QUALEFFO)	**Lips P et al.** Quality of life in patients with vertebral fractures: validation of the Quality of Life Questionnaire of the European Foundation for Osteoporosis (QUALEFFO). *Osteoporosis international*, 1999, **10**:150–160.
Quality of Life Scale	**Leedham B et al.** Positive expectations predict health after heart transplantation. *Health psychology*, 1995, **14**:74–69.
Quality of Life Time Trade Off	**Torrance GW.** Social preferences for health status: an empirical evaluation of three measurement techniques. *Socio-economic planning sciences*, 1976, **10**:129–136.
Quality of Life — 15-Dimensional Measure	**Sintonen H, Pekurinen M.** A fifteen dimensional measure of health-related quality of life and its applications. In: Walker SR, Rosser RM, eds. *Quality of life assessment: key issues in the 1990's.* Dordrecht, The Netherlands, Kluwer Academic, 1990:185–195.
Quality of Life — Hip Replacement	**Cleary PD et al.** Using patient reports to assess health related quality of life after total hip replacement. *Quality of life research*, 1993, **2**:3–11.
Quality of Well Being	**Kaplan RM, Bush JW, Berry CC.** The reliability, stability and generalizability of a health status index. *Proceedings of the social statistics sections.* American Statistical Association, 1978:704–709.
	Kaplan RM, Bush JW. Health-related quality of life measurement for evaluation, research and policy analyses. *Health psychology*, 1982, **1**:61–80.
Quality of Well-Being Scale — Version 6B	**Anderson JP.** Quality of Well-Being Scale — Version 6B. San Diego, CA, Health Policy Project M-022, University of California San Diego, 1989.
Rand Health Insurance Study Scale (HIS) — Children	**Eisen M, Ware JE, Donald D.** Measuring components of children's health status. *Medical care*, 1979, **17**:902–921.
Rapid Disability Rating Scale (RDRS)	**Linn MW.** A Rapid Disability Rating Scale. *Journal of the American Geriatrics Society*, 1967, **15**:211–214.
Rapid Disability Rating Scale — 2 (RDRS-2)	**Linn MW, Linn BS.** The Rapid Disability Rating Scale-2. *Journal of the American Geriatrics Society*, 1982, **30**:378–382.
Rheumatoid Arthritis Disease Activity Index (RADAI)	**Stucki G et al.** A self-administered Rheumatoid Arthritis Disease Activity Index (RADAI) for epidemiologic research. *Arthritis and rheumatism*, 1995, **38**:795–798.

Table 32 (*Continued*)

Instrument	Citations[a]
Rheumatoid Arthritis Patient's Questionnaire	**Riemsma RP et al.** Coordinated individual education with an arthritis passport for patients with rheumatoid arthritis. *Arthritis care and research*, 1997, **10**:238–249.
Rheumatoid Arthritis-Specific Quality of Life Instrument (RAQoL)	**DeJong Z et al.** The reliability and construct validity of the RAQoL: a rheumatoid arthritis-specific quality of life instrument. *British journal of rheumatology*, 1997, **36**:878–883.
Risk Factor Questionnaire (RFQ) Perceived Workload Assessment	**Halpern M et al.** The test-retest of a new questionnaire for outcome studies of low back pain. *Applied ergonomics*, 2001, **32**:39–46.
Roland Scale	**Roland M, Morris R.** A study of the natural history of back pain. I. Development of a reliable and sensitive measure of disability in low-back pain. *Spine*, 1983, **3**:141–144.
Rosser Disability/Distress Scale	**Rosser R, Watts V.** The measurement of illness. *Journal of the operational research society*, 1978, **29**:529. **Rosser RM, Kind P.** A scale of valuation states of illness: is there a social consensus? *International journal of epidemiology*, 1978, **7**:347–358.
Schober-Modified-Modified	**Williams R et al.** Reliability of the modified-modified Schober and double inclinometer methods for measuring lumbar flexion and extension. *Physical therapy*, 1993, **73**:33–44.
Scoliosis Research Society Outcomes Instrument for Adolescents	**Hahrer TR et al.** *Results of the Scoliosis Research Society Instrument for evaluation of surgical outcome in adolescent idiopathic scoliosis: a multi-center study of 244 patients*. New York, NY, St Vincent's Hospital Medical Center, Department of Orthopaedic Surgery, 1998.
Self-Evaluation of Life Function Scale (SELF) — Older Adults	**Linn MW, Linn RS.** Self-Evaluation of Life Function (SELF) Scale: a comprehensive self-report of health for elderly adults. *Journal of gerontology*, 1984, **39**:603–612.
Self-Evaluation of Life Function Scale — "Abbreviated" — Older Adults	**Rapkin BD, Fisher K.** Framing the construct of life satisfaction in terms of older adults' personal goals. *Psychology and aging*, 1992, **7**:138–149.
Self-Evaluation Scales for ADLS (SESA)	**Nojima Y et al.** Perception of time among Japanese inpatients. *Western journal of nursing research*, 1987, **9**:288–300.
SF-36 (Short Form Health Status Survey)	**Ware JE, Sherbourne CD.** The MOS 36-Item Short Form Health Status Survey (SF-36). 1. Conception framework and item selection. *Medical care*, 1992, **30**:473–483.
Short Arthritis Impact Measurement Scales (SAIMS)	**Wallston KA et al.** Comparing the short and long versions of the Arthritis Impact Measurement Scales. *Journal of rheumatology*, 1989, **16**:1105–1109.
Shoulder Pain and Disability Index	**Roach KE et al.** Development of a Shoulder Pain and Disability Index. *Arthritis care research*, 1991, **4**:143–149.
Sickness Impact Profile (SIP)	**Bergner M et al.** The Sickness Impact Profile: development and final revision of a health status measure. *Medical care*, 1981, **19**:787–805.

Table 32 (*Continued*)

Instrument	Citations[a]
Stulberg Classification System	**Neyt JG et al.** Stulberg Classification System for evaluation of Legg-Calve-Perthes Disease: intra-rater and inter-rater reliability. *Journal of bone and joint surgery*. 1999, **81**:1209–1216.
Swedish Health-Related Quality of Life Survey (SWED QUAL)	**Brorsson B, Ifver J, Hays RD.** The Swedish Health-Related Quality of Life Survey (SWED-QUAL). *Quality of life research*, 1993, **2**:33–45.
Time Trade-off Utility	**Torrance GW, Thomas WH, Sackett DL.** A utility maximization model for evaluation of health care programs. *Health services research*, 1972, **7**:118.
Toronto Functional Capacity Questionnaire	**Helewa A, Goldsmith CH, Smyth HA.** Independent measurement of functional capacity in rheumatoid arthritis. *Journal of rheumatology*, 1982, **9**:794–797.
Total Hip Arthroplasty Outcome Evaluation Form	**Liang MH et al.** The American Academy of Orthopaedic Surgeons Task Force on Outcomes Studies. The total hip arthroplasty outcome evaluation form of the American Academy of Orthopaedic Surgeons. *Journal of bone and joint surgery*, 1991, **73**:639–646.
Tufts Assessment of Motor Performance (TAMP)	**Ludlow LH, Haley SM, Gans BM.** A hierarchical model of functional performance in rehabilitation medicine: the Tufts Assessment of Motor Performance. *Evaluation and the health professions*, 1992, **15**:59–74.
	Haley SM et al. Tufts Assessment of Motor Performance. *Archives of physical medicine and rehabilitation*, 1991, **72**:359–366.
	Gans BM et al. Description and interobserver reliability of the Tufts Assessment of Motor Performance. *American journal of physical medicine and rehabilitation*, 1988, **67**:202–210.
U-Titer	**Sumner W et al.** U-Titer: a utility assessment tool. *Medical decision making*, 1991, **11**:327.
	Nease RF Jr et al. Automated utility assessment of global health. *Quality of life research*, 1996, **5**:175–182.
Utility Measure	**Katz JN et al.** Stability and responsiveness of utility measures. *Medical care*, 1994, **32**:183–188.
Utility Measures for Quality of Life	**Torrance GW.** Utility approach to measuring health-related quality of life. *Journal of chronic diseases*, 1987, **40**:593–600.
Vigor Questionnaire	**Keating EM, Ranawat CS, Cats-Baril W.** Assessment of postoperative vigor in patients undergoing elective total joint arthroplasty: a concise patient-and caregiver-based instrument. *Orthopedics*, 1999, **22** (suppl. 1):119–128.
Waddell Signs	**Waddell G et al.** Nonorganic physical signs in low back pain. *Spine*, 1980, **5**:117–125.
Western Ontario and McMaster Universities Osteoarthritis Index (WOMAC)	**Bellamy N et al.** Validation Study of WOMAC: a health status instrument for measuring clinically important patient relevant outcomes to anti-rheumatic drug therapy in patients with osteoarthritis of the hip or knee. *Journal of rheumatology*, 1988, **15**:1833–1840.

Table 32 (*Continued*)

Instrument	Citations[a]
	Bellamy N et al. Validation study of WOMAC: a health status instrument for measuring clinically important patient relevant outcomes following total hip or knee arthroplasty in osteoarthritis. *Journal of orthopedics and rheumatology*, 1988, **1**:95–108.
World Health Organization Disability Assessment Schedule (WHODAS II)	*WHO Psychiatric Disability Assessment Schedule (WHO/DAS).* Geneva, World Health Organization, 1988.
World Health Organization Quality of Life (WHOQOL)	Study protocol for the World Health Organization project to develop a Quality of Life assessment instrument (WHOQOL). *Quality of life research*, 1993, **2**:153–159.
Workplace Medical Examination Form (WMEF)	Harwood KJ et al. Low back pain assessment training of industry-based physicians. *Journal of rehabilitation*, 1997, **34**:371–382. Campello M et al. Approaches to improve the outcome of patients with delayed recovery. *Baillière's clinical rheumatology*, 1997, **12**:93–11.

[a] These citations describe the characteristics, reliability and validity for each instrument. If it was not possible to obtain the original reference, a secondary source was used. In some instances additional citations were given because all relevant information was not included in the first citation.

9. Conclusions and recommendations

Musculoskeletal disorders are the most frequent causes of physical disability, at least in developed countries. As mortality from infectious diseases reduces worldwide, the global population is ageing and the numbers of people in the oldest age groups are increasing. As the prevalence of many musculoskeletal disorders increases with age, the likely result is that there will be a growth in the number of people with chronic disabling disorders. It follows that there will be a marked increase in requirements for health care and community support in the coming years. Moreover, musculoskeletal traumas, particularly those caused by road accidents, are a major cause of both mortality and chronic impairment in people of all ages, especially the young and productive.

Clearly, it is desirable to alter the predicted increase in the number of persons suffering from musculoskeletal conditions and the subsequent disabilities affecting both the physical and the psychological domains. In order to be able to change priorities and develop preventive strategies, it is essential to possess accurate data on the present situation. Furthermore, in order to be able to measure the results of interventions, it is necessary to have baseline information not only on incidence and prevalence but also on the effects on individuals and society.

This report describes what is known in terms of both numbers and different outcome or impact estimates. It is also the first effort to summarize comprehensively the effect of all major musculoskeletal conditions. An attempt has been made to find common features instead of pointing out differences. However, successful treatment of the individual patient relies on multidisciplinary care.

This approach also allows comparison with other diseases. First, however, it is necessary to define and agree on the most useful measures for describing the burden.

9.1 Incidence and prevalence

The first step is to obtain an accurate estimate of the number of people currently suffering from musculoskeletal conditions, taking into account global and geographical differences. It is clearly more difficult to make estimates for non-fatal outcomes than for fatal ones, as this requires an understanding of the natural history of the condition. Musculoskeletal conditions may have either an acute or a gradual onset. Their outcomes vary from complete restoration of health to a chronic progressive course. A wrist fracture, for example, has an acute onset but may heal completely without any further complaints, whereas osteoarthritis has an insidious onset and may or may not progress to total joint stiffness. The consequence of this variability is that incidence is the most relevant measure for some conditions, whereas prevalence is the only measure available for others.

The Scientific Group therefore agreed that certain basic requirements were necessary to access data that can be compared across musculoskeletal conditions:

— agreed definitions of each condition to be used in all future studies;
— agreed age bands for reporting data or available as raw data;
— reported data separated by gender;
— guidelines for the uniform collection of data.

In addition it became obvious that data were lacking for almost all conditions in certain parts of the world, particularly Africa, South America and Eastern Europe. However, it was pointed out that it might be possible to extrapolate from one region to another that was economically and culturally similar, while recognizing the limitations of doing so in connection with global calculations of disease burden.

Furthermore, the possibility was recognized that certain sources of existing data were not being fully utilized, such as government surveys, health care and pension funds, and government providers (hospital discharge data, emergency room registrations, etc.).

9.2 Severity and course of the conditions

Musculoskeletal conditions may be severely incapacitating, but they may also heal with or without sequelae and with or without treatment. The course of these conditions is not always predictable, although certain patterns predominate. With a view to enhancing comparability, the group reached agreement on the most relevant model for the course of each condition by assigning stages and levels of severity.

9.2.1 *Rheumatoid arthritis*

For rheumatoid arthritis the currently used Steinbrocker's functional capacity and radiographic assessment has significant limitations. The following categories should therefore be considered for staging rheumatoid arthritis: degree of inflammation, structural damage, clinical damage, function, and severity of clinical outlook.

9.2.2 *Osteoarthritis*

For osteoarthritis a definition based on symptoms was recommended: osteoarthritis is a condition characterized by use-related joint pain experienced on most days in any given month, for which no other cause is apparent.

Staging in accordance with X-ray findings is commonly used. However, the value of this method has limitations because X-ray findings are not directly transferable to subjective symptoms or physical findings. Furthermore, X-rays are not widely available in all parts of the world, so symptomatic or physical staging has additional advantages.

9.2.3 *Osteoporosis*

Osteoporosis may be divided into two stages:

1. A bone mineral density T-score of less than –2.5 without fracture, i.e. an asymptomatic stage.

2. Fragility fractures and the post-fracture stage: the fracture stage may start with a fracture at various sites, in various sequences, and the number of fractures may accumulate.

9.2.4 *Spinal disorders*

Spinal disorders pose difficulties because nonspecific spinal disorders account for 80% of the cases seen. The recommended staging system should combine duration, symptoms, functional status, physical findings and radiographic data, but there should also be a simplified form employing clinical data only when X-rays are not available. A four-step grading system, from mild to severe, was regarded as being the most appropriate.

9.2.5 *Severe limb trauma*

Because of the acute onset, severe limb trauma does not entirely fit a model developed for chronic progressive conditions. The severity of limb trauma is generally characterized by:

— the location of the injury;
— the type and extent of bone injury, for example the type of fracture and the extent of bone loss;
— the extent of soft tissue damage, such as muscle or tendon damage, the size of the skin defect, and any neurovascular damage.

Existing classification systems recognize these assessments and should be more widely used. These systems are, however, based on the acute evaluation of the extent of the injury, whereas the duration of impairment and the long-term functional outcome need to be correlated and validated against these measures.

9.3 Health and economic indicators

It may be useful to regard health as a multidimensional function. Consequently, a lack of full health is incompletely described by a diagnosis, which health care providers have traditionally found to be satisfactory for categorizing patients. A loss of health may be more satisfactorily described as disability and a loss of function, including a loss of bodily functional ability, a loss of the capacity to carry out tasks as an individual and a loss of functioning or an inability to participate in society. Adaptation and coping should also be considered to be factors that profoundly affect the ultimate outcome, i.e. well-being and the quality of life. Various indicators of health can be used to describe this from the perspective of the person with the health condition, the carers, the providers or the state.

Economic indicators are similarly related to the person suffering or to society. As each society has limited resources for health care, and as these resources are generated by the people constituting the society, increased or decreased spending on musculoskeletal conditions by the health care system affects the care of individual patients. For these conditions the direct cost varies from 10% to 40% of the total expenditure. Consequently, commonly used indices such as the use of hospital beds are less relevant than measures of indirect costs such as the number of work days lost or the inability to secure life support. Furthermore, the economic indicators must be adjusted for geographical and cultural differences.

9.4 Measuring health impact and economic burden at the population level

The impact at population level can be assessed through various surveys, either for a certain condition or for musculoskeletal conditions in general. The common agreed indicators were:

- pain related to the musculoskeletal system, bones and joints;
- limited mobility;
- the ability to perform activities of daily living;
- limited participation in society because of musculoskeletal complaints.

Specific population studies can assess risk factors for the development and progression of conditions. This makes it possible to create preventive strategies. At the population level, complaints related to musculoskeletal conditions can be expressed in monetary terms. The direct cost or medical expenditure may be assessed by reference to indicators such as the number of visits to outpatient clinics, the number of hospital admissions, laboratory and imaging procedures, the rehabilitation service and durable medical equipment.

The indirect costs may be assessed by indicators such as loss of work and the expenditure of work compensation programmes. Such estimates, however, are subject to a relatively high degree of unreliability as the models are, to some extent, based on assumptions. For example, it may be assumed that there is unpaid support from family members. It also has to be recognized that many indicators cannot be used globally because of differences in the organization of health care systems and in the availability of care. It is therefore necessary to identify simple indicators that can be used universally.

9.5 Describing health status as a consequence of illness or injury: impact on the individual

Measures of health status provide information on a variety of domains that represent health. Combinations of domains tested through specific and validated questions comprise the numerous assessment instruments that are available. The advantage of using generic instruments is that comparability is achieved with conditions outside the musculoskeletal field. However, a disadvantage lies in the choice of relevant domains included in a particular instrument i.e. in the sensitivity to musculoskeletal conditions. Disease-specific instruments, on the other hand, may only allow comparison of the health status of a specific condition either cross-sectionally between centres or longitudinally, e.g. following new treatments.

Of a set of core domains and subdomains the Scientific Group viewed the following as being the most relevant for musculoskeletal conditions:

— physical health, with subdomains, and pain and physical function (mobility and activities of daily living);
— social health;
— mental health, with subdomains, and energy/vitality and anxiety.

The most useful generic and specific instruments considered for each condition are presented in Table 33. None of the measures captures all the important dimensions with sufficient depth to fully characterize the impact of each condition. However, for the purposes of broad, population-based monitoring, it was considered essential to choose brief, practical measures that could be translated across many different cultures.

The evaluation of children's health status necessitates additional considerations because not only the children but also their family units are affected. The applicability of the health domains to the child–family unit therefore has to be addressed, and the specific problems of development and growth have to be accounted for. The tools available all have limited applicability here.

9.6 Recommendations of the Scientific Group

- Guidelines should be developed to facilitate the uniform collection of data for comparison between geographical regions and longitudinal assessment of changes in disease patterns.
- The most essential regions from which data are missing should be identified in order to obtain a true global picture of the frequency with which common musculoskeletal conditions occur.
- It is necessary to develop and validate simple instruments in a format that can be used worldwide in order to measure the impact of musculoskeletal conditions on health and economies, both on individuals and on society.
- Agreement on definition and staging of musculoskeletal conditions is essential, as indicated in the report.

In order to assess the health impact on the individual, it may be of help to ascribe health states by evaluating the most important domains of life affected by the condition in question. For all musculoskeletal conditions, pain and mobility are considered to be the most

Table 33
The most relevant instruments for musculoskeletal conditions

Musculoskeletal conditions	Instruments	
	Generic	Disease-specific
Rheumatoid arthritis	Short Form Health Status Survey (SF-36)	Arthritis Impact Measurement Scale-2 (AIMS-2) Rheumatic Arthritis Patient Questionnaire
Osteoarthritis, lower limb	WHO Disability Assessment Schedule (WHODAS II) SF-36	Western Ontario and McMaster Universities Osteoarthritis Index (WOMAC) AIMS-2 Disease Repercussion Profile (DRP)
Osteoarthritis, upper limb	WHODAS II SF-36	Australian/Canadian Osteoarthritis Hand Index (AUSCAN) AAOS Disabilities of the Arm, Shoulder and Hand Instrument (DASH) DRP
Osteoporosis	Nottingham Health Profile (NHP) SF-36 EuroQol (EQ-5D)	Quality of Life Questionnaire of the European Foundation for Osteoporosis (Qualeffo-41) Osteoporosis Assessment Questionnaire (OPAQ)
Spinal disorders	SF-36	Oswestry Roland Kohlmann–Raspe
Severe limb trauma	SF-36	Musculoskeletal Functional Assessment (MFA)
Conditions specific to children		Pediatric Evaluation of Disability Inventory (PEDI) Child Health Questionnaire (CHQ)

important domains. The instruments available for measuring impact and outcome are identified, and the most widely used or most valuable instruments, both generic and specific, are defined, although none is currently regarded as being truly optimal.

ACKNOWLEDGEMENTS

The Scientific Group gratefully acknowledges the contribution made to the organization of the meeting by members Professor A.D. Woolf (Chairman, editor), Dr K. Åkesson (Joint Vice-Chairman, co-editor), Professor J.M. Hazes (Joint

Vice-Chairman, co-editor), Professor B. Browner, Professor M. Cimmino, Professor C. Cooper, Professor F. Guillemin, Professor M. Hochberg, Dr C. Shewan, Professor G. Stucki, Professor D. Symmons, Professor S. van der Linden, Professor N. Walsh and WHO Geneva, Switzerland, staff members Dr A. Lopez, Dr R. Lozano and Dr T.B. Üston.

The Scientific Group also acknowledges the contributions made to the preparation of the Technical Report by the chairs and organizers of the meeting, by the rapporteurs and by Professor N. Bellamy, Professor P. Brooks, Dr L. Callahan, Professor O. Johnell, Professor J. Kanis, Professor H. Raspe and Professor R. Rizzoli.

The Scientific Group wishes to acknowledge the important academic contributions received from a wide range of experts from different countries who provided data on the burden of musculoskeletal conditions, as well as the support in data collation and preparation of the contents of the Technical Report given by Scientific Group member Ms D. Pattison, Dr S. Lybrand, Royal Brisbane Hospital, Brisbane, Queensland, Australia, and Dr B. Pfleger, WHO, Geneva, Switzerland.

The Scientific Group wishes to acknowledge the organizational and financial support of the Bone and Joint Decade.

References

1. *Assessment of fracture risk and its application to screening for postmenopausal osteoporosis. Report of a WHO Study Group.* Geneva, World Health Organization, 1994 (WHO Technical Report Series, No. 843).
2. World Bank. *World development report 1993. Investing in health.* New York, Oxford University Press, 1993.
3. Lozano R et al. Burden of disease assessment and health system reform: results of a study in Mexico. *Journal for international development*, 1995, 7:555–564.
4. *The world health report 2000. Health systems: improving performance.* Geneva, World Health Organization, 2000.
5. Murray CJL, Lopez AD, eds. *The global burden of disease: a comprehensive assessment of mortality and disability from diseases, injuries and risk factors in 1990 and projected to 2020.* Cambridge, MA, Harvard University Press, 1996 (Global Burden of Disease and Injury Series, Vol. 1).
6. *National burden of disease studies: a practical guide.* Global programme on evidence for health policy. Geneva, World Health Organization, 2001.
7. Weiser S. Psychosocial aspects of occupational musculoskeletal disorders. In: Nordin M, Andersson GBJ, Pope MH, eds. *Musculoskeletal disorders in the workplace: principles and practices.* Philadelphia, CV Mosby, 1997:51–56.
8. Arnett FC et al. The American Rheumatism Association 1987 revised criteria for the classification of rheumatoid arthritis. *Arthritis and rheumatism*, 1988, 30:315–324.
9. Ramsey SE et al. Comparison of criteria for the classification of childhood arthritis. *Journal of rheumatology*, 2000, 27:1283–1286.

10. **Abdel-Nasser AM, Rasker JJ, Valkenburg HA.** Epidemiological and clinical aspects relating to the variability of rheumatoid arthritis. *Seminars in arthritis and rheumatism* 1997, **27**:123–140.

11. **Spector TD, Hart DJ, Powell RJ.** Prevalence of rheumatoid arthritis and rheumatoid factor in women: evidence for a secular decline. *Annals of the rheumatic diseases*, 1993, **52**:54–57.

12. **Silman AJ et al.** Absence of rheumatoid arthritis in a rural Nigerian population. *Journal of rheumatology*, 1993, **20**:618–622.

13. **Symmons D, Harrison B.** Early inflammatory polyarthritis: results from the Norfolk Arthritis Register with a review of the literature. I. Risk factors for the development of inflammatory polyarthritis and rheumatoid arthritis. *Rheumatology*, 2000, **39**:835–843.

14. **Lawrence JS, Bremner JM, Bier F.** Osteoarthrosis prevalence in the population and the relationship between symptoms and X-ray changes. *Annals of the rheumatic diseases*, 1966, **25**:1–24.

15. **Dieppe P.** What is the relationship between pain and osteoarthritis? *Rheumatology in Europe*, 1998, **27**:55–56.

16. **Altman R et al.** The American College of Rheumatology criteria for the classification and reporting of osteoarthritis of the hand. *Arthritis and rheumatism*, 1990, **33**:1601–1610.

17. **Altman R et al.** The American College of Rheumatology criteria for the classification and reporting of osteoarthritis of the hip. *Arthritis and rheumatism*, 1991, **34**:505–514.

18. **Altman R et al.** Development of criteria for the classification and reporting of osteoarthritis: classification of osteoarthritis of the knee. *Arthritis and rheumatism*, 1986, **29**:1039–1049.

19. **Mathers C, Vos T, Stevenson C.** *The burden of disease and injury in Australia.* Canberra, Australian Institute of Health and Welfare, 1999 (AIHW Catalogue No. PHE 17).

20. **van Saase JLCM et al.** Epidemiology of osteoarthritis: Zoetermeer survey. Comparison of radiological osteoarthritis in a Dutch population with that in 10 other populations. *Annals of the rheumatic diseases*, 1989, **48**:271–280.

21. **Skinner TJ, ed.** *The national health survey: summary of results. Australian edition.* Canberra, Australian Bureau of Statistics, 1995 (ABS Catalogue No. 4364.0).

22. **Hill CL et al.** Health related quality of life in a population sample with arthritis. *Journal of rheumatology*, 1999, **26**:2029–2035.

23. **Garden RS.** Stability and union in subcapital fractures of the femur. *Journal of bone and joint surgery*, 1964, **46-B**:630–647.

24. **Ettinger B et al.** Reduction of vertebral fracture risk in postmenopausal women with osteoporosis treated with raloxifene. *Journal of the American Medical Association*, 1999, **282**:637–645.

25. **van Staa TP et al.** Epidemiology of fractures in England and Wales. *Bone*, 2001, **29**:517–522.

26. **Oleksik A et al.** Health-related quality of life in postmenopausal women with low BMD with or without prevalent vertebral fractures. *Journal of bone and mineral research*, 2000, **15**:1384–1392.

27. **Glorieux FH, Karsenty G, Thakker RV.** Metabolic bone disease in children: rickets and osteomalacia. In: Avioli LV, Krane SM, eds. *Metabolic bone disease*, 3rd ed. Boston, MA, Academic Press, 1998:759–783.

28. **Parfitt AM.** Osteomalacia and related disorders. In: Avioli LV and Krane SM, eds. *Metabolic bone disease*, 3rd ed. Academic Press, Boston, MA, 1998:328–386.

29. **Kanis JA et al.** Long-term risk of osteoporotic fracture in Malmo. *Osteoporosis international*, 2000, **11**:669–674.

30. **Cooper C, Campion G, Melton LJ III.** Hip fractures in the elderly: a world-wide projection. *Osteoporosis international*, 1992, **2**:285–289.

31. **Kanis JA et al.** International variations in hip fracture probabilities: implications for risk assessment. *Journal of bone and mineral research*, 2002, **17**:1237–1244.

32. **Gullberg B, Johnell O, Kanis JA.** World-wide projections for hip fracture. *Osteoporosis international*, 1997, **7**:407–413.

33. **Johnell O et al.** The apparent incidence of hip fracture in Europe: a study of national register sources: the MEDOS Study Group. *Osteoporosis international*, 1992, **2**:298–302.

34. Incidence of vertebral fracture in Europe: results from the European Prospective Osteoporosis Study (EPOS). *Journal of bone and mineral research*, 2002, **17**:716–724.

35. **Van der Klift M et al.** The incidence of vertebral fractures in men and women: the Rotterdam Study. *Journal of bone and mineral research*, 2002, **17**:1051–1056.

36. **Melton LJ III et al.** Perspective. How many women have osteoporosis? *Journal of bone and mineral research*, 1992, **7**:1005–1010.

37. **Johnell O, Gullberg B, Kanis JA.** The hospital burden of vertebral fracture in Europe: a study of National Register sources. *Osteoporosis international*, 1997, **7**:138–144.

38. **Bengner U, Johnell O.** Increasing incidence of forearm fractures. A comparison of epidemiologic patterns 25 years apart. *Acta orthopaedica Scandinavica*, 1985, **56**:158–160.

39. **O'Neill TW et al.** Incidence of distal forearm fracture in British men and women. *Osteoporosis international*, 2001, **12**:555–558.

40. **Kanis JA et al.** The burden of osteoporotic fractures: a method for setting intervention thresholds. *Osteoporosis international*, 2001, **12**:417–427.

41. **SBU The Swedish Council on Technology Assessment in Health Care.** Measuring bone mineral density. Stockholm, 1995 (SBU Report 127).

42. **Kanis JA, Gluer CC, Committee of Scientific Advisors of the IOF.** An update on the diagnosis and assessment of osteoporosis with densitometry. *Osteoporosis international*, 2000, **11**:192–202.

43. **Kanis JA et al.** Risk of hip fracture according to the WHO criteria for osteopenia and osteoporosis. *Bone*, 2000, **27**:585–590.

44. **Holick MF.** Vitamin D: new horizons for the 21st century. *American journal of clinical nutrition*, 1994, **60**:619–630.

45. **Feleke Y et al.** Low levels of serum calcidiol in an African population compared to a North European population. *European journal of endocrinology*, 1999, **141**:358–360.

46. **Marie PJ et al.** Histological osteomalacia due to dietary calcium deficiency in children. *New England journal of medicine*, 1982, **307**:584–588.

47. **Sedrani SH, Elidrissy AWTH, El Arabi KM.** Sunlight and vitamin D status in normal Saudi subjects. *American journal of clinical nutrition*, 1983, **38**:129–132.

48. **Bettica P et al.** High prevalence of hypovitaminosis D among free-living postmenopausal women referred to an osteoporosis outpatient clinic in northern Italy for initial screening. *Osteoporosis international*, 1999, **9**:226–229.

49. **Lips P, Obrant KJ.** The pathogenesis and treatment of hip fractures. *Osteoporosis international*, 1991, **1**:218–231.

50. **Lips P.** Vitamin D deficiency and secondary hyperparathyroidism in the elderly. Consequences for bone loss and fractures and therapeutic implications. *Endocrine reviews,* 2001, **22**:477–501.

51. **Borenstein DG, Wiesel SW.** *Low back pain: medical diagnosis and comprehensive management.* Philadelphia, PA, WB Saunders, 1989.

52. **White AA III, Gordon SL.** Synopsis: workshop on idiopathic low-back pain. *Spine*, 1982, **7**:141–149.

53. **Nachemson AL, Jonsson EJ.** *Neck and back pain. The scientific evidence of causes, diagnoses and treatment.* Philadelphia, PA, Lippincott Williams and Wilkins, 2000:241–304.

54. **Spitzer WO et al.** Scientific approach to the assessment and management of activity-related spinal disorders: report of the Quebec Task Force on Spinal Disease. *Spine*, 1987, **12**(suppl. 7):1–59.

55. **Frymoyer JW.** Epidemiology, magnitude of the problem. In: Wienstein JN, Weisel SW, eds. *The lumbar spine: the International Society for the Study of the Lumbar Spine.* Philadelphia, PA, WB Saunders, 1990:32–38.

56. **Biering-Sorenson F.** Low back trouble in a general population of 30-, 40-, 50- and 60-year-old men and women: study design, representativeness and basic results. *Danish medical bulletin*, 1982, **29**:289–299.

57. **Barnsley L, Lord S, Bogduk N.** The pathophysiology of whiplash. *Spine: state of the art reviews*, 1993, **7**:329–353.

58. **Carey TS et al.** The outcomes and cost of care for acute low back pain among patients seen by primary care practitioners, chiropractors and orthopedic surgeons. *New England journal of medicine*, 1995, **333**:913–917.

59. **Von Korff M.** Studying the natural history of low back pain. *Spine*, 1993, **19**(suppl. 18):2041–2046.

60. **Deyo RA, Tsui-Wu YJ.** Descriptive epidemiology of low back pain and its related medical care in the United States. *Spine*, 1987, **12**:264–268.

61. **Hurwitz EL, Morgenstern H.** Correlates of back problems and back-related disability in the United States. *Journal of clinical epidemiology*, 1997, **50**:669–681.

62. **Edwards S.** *Evaluation of the National Health Interview Survey diagnostic reporting*. Rockville, MD, Westat, 1992 (Report to National Center for Health Care Statistics).

63. **Andersson GBJ.** The epidemiology of spinal disorders. In: Frymoyer JW, ed. *The adult spine: principles and practice*. Philadelphia, PA, Lippincott-Raven, 1997:93–141.

64. **Pope MH, Frymoyer JW, Andersson GBJ.** *Occupational low back pain*. New York, NY, Praeger, 1984.

65. **Riksforsakringsverket [National Office of Social Security].** *Statistical information Is-1, 1987–8*. Stockholm, 1987–1988.

66. **Valkenburg HA, Haanen HCM.** The epidemiology of low back pain. In: White AA, Gordon SL, eds. *Symposium on idiopathic low back pain*. St Louis, MO, CV Mosby, 1982:9–22.

67. **Mulimba JO.** The problems of low back pain in Africa. *East African medical journal*, 1990, **67**:250–253.

68. **Loney PD, Stratford PW.** The prevalence of low back pain in adults: a methodological review of the literature. *Physical therapy*, 1999, **79**:384–396.

69. **National Research Council and Institute of Medicine.** *Musculoskeletal disorders and the workplace: low back and upper extremities*. Washington, DC, National Academy Press, 2001 (available at: http://www.nap.edu).

70. **Volinn E.** The epidemiology of low back pain in the rest of the world. *Spine*, 1997, **22**:1747–1754.

71. **Walker BF.** The prevalence of low back pain: a systematic review of the literature from 1966 to 1998. *Journal of spinal disorders*, 2000, **13**:205–217.

72. **Adams PF, Hendershot, GE, Maranao MA.** *Current estimates, from the National Health Interview Survey, 1996*. Hyattsville, MD, National Center for Health Statistics, 1999 (Vital and Health Statistics Series 10, No. 200. DHHS Publication No. [PHS] 99–1528) (available at: *http://www.cdc.gov/nchs/data/series/sr_10/sr10_200.pdf*).

73. **Agency for Healthcare Research and Quality.** *Nationwide inpatient sample*. Rockville, MD, 2000 (available at: http://www.ahrq.gov/data/hcup/hcupnis.htm).

74. **Mock CN et al.** Incidence and outcome of injury in Ghana: results of a community based survey. *Bulletin of the World Health Organization*, 1999, **77**:955–964.

75. **Murray CJL, Lopez AD.** *Global health statistics*. Geneva, World Health Organization, 1996 (Global Burden of Disease and Injury Series, Vol. II).

76. **Chopra A et al.** Prevalence of rheumatic diseases in a rural population in western India: a WHO–ILAR COPCORD study. *Journal of the Association of Physicians of India*, 2001, **49**:240–246.

77. **Steinbrocker O, Traeger CH, Batterman RC.** Therapeutic criteria in rheumatoid arthritis. *Journal of the American Medical Association*, 1949, **140**:659.

78. **Cimmino MA et al.** Extraarticular manifestations in 587 Italian patients with rheumatoid arthritis. *Rheumatology international*, 2000, **19**:213–217.

79. **Guillemin F, Bombardier C, Beaton D.** Cross-cultural adaptation of health-related quality of life measures: literature review and proposed guidelines. *Journal of clinical epidemiology*, 1993, **46**:1417–1432.

80. **Spiegel TM, Spiegel JS, Paulus HE.** The joint alignment and motion scale: a simple measure of deformity in patients with rheumatoid arthritis. *Journal of rheumatology*, 1987, **14**:887–892.

81. **Mathers C, Penm R.** *Health system costs of injury, poisoning and musculoskeletal disorders in Australia 1993–94.* Canberra, Australian Institute of Health and Welfare, 1999 (AIHW Catalogue No. HWE 12; Health and Welfare Expenditure Series No. 6).

82. **Pluijm SM et al.** Consequences of vertebral deformities in older men and women. *Journal of bone and mineral research*, 2000, **15**:1564–1572.

83. **Oleksik AM et al.** Three years of health-related quality of life assessment in postmenopausal women with osteoporosis: impact of incident vertebral fractures, age and severe adverse events. *Journal of bone and mineral research*, 2000, **15**(suppl. 1):S168.

84. **Hunt S, McEwen J, McKenna SP.** Measuring health status: a new tool for clinicians and epidemiologists. *Journal of the Royal College of General Practitioners*, 1985, **35**:185–188.

85. **Ware JE, Kosinski M, Keller SD.** *SF-36 physical and mental health summary scales: a user's manual.* Boston, MA, The New England Medical Center, 1994.

86. **Van Agt HM et al.** Test–retest reliability of health state valuations collected with the EuroQol questionnaire. *Social science and medicine*, 1994, **39**:1537–1544.

87. **Lips P et al.** Quality of life in patients with vertebral fractures: validation of the Quality of Life Questionnaire of the European Foundation for Osteoporosis (QUALEFFO). *Osteoporosis international*, 1999, **10**:150–160.

88. **Randell AG et al.** Quality of life in osteoporosis: reliability, consistency and validity of the Osteoporosis Assessment Questionnaire. *Journal of rheumatology*, 1998, **25**:1171–1179.

89. **Cook DJ et al.** Measuring quality of life in women with osteoporosis. *Osteoporosis international*, 1997, **7**:478–487.

90. **Chandler JM et al.** Reliability of an Osteoporosis-Targeted Quality of Life survey instrument for use in the community: OPTQoL. *Osteoporosis international*, 1998, **8**:127–135.

91. **Dolan P, Torgerson D, Kumar Kakarlapadi T.** Health-related quality of life in Colles' fracture patients. *Osteoporosis international*, 1999, **9**:196–199.

92. **Nevitt MC et al.** The association of radiographically detected vertebral fractures with back pain and function: a prospective study. *Annals of internal medicine*, 1998, **128**:793–800.

93. **Cooper C.** The crippling consequences of fractures and their impact on quality of life. *American journal of medicine*, 1997, **103**:12S–19S.

94. **Lesnyak O, Kuzmina L, Lesnyak Y.** Social impact of hip fractures in elderly in Russia. *Osteoporosis international*, 2000, **11**(suppl. 5):S4.

95. **Waddell G.** Biophysical analysis of low back pain. *Baillière's clinical rheumatology*, 1992, **6**:523–557.

96. **Von Korff M.** Studying the natural history of low back pain. *Spine*, 1993, **19**(suppl. 18):2041–2046.

97. **Weinstein JN, Gordon SL.** *Low back pain: a scientific and clinical review.* Rosemont, IL, American Academy of Orthopaedic Surgeons, 1996.

98. **Harris Poll.** *Survey of pain in the United States of America: the Nuprin Pain Report.* Somerville, NJ, Bristol-Meyers, 1985.

99. **Reisbord LS, Greenland S.** Factors associated with self-reported back pain prevalence: a population based study. *Journal of chronic disease*, 1985, **38**:691–702.

100. **Bigos SJ et al.** *Acute low back problems in adults.* Rockville, MD, Agency for Health Care Policy and Research, Public Health Service, United States Department of Health and Human Services, 1994 (AHCPR publication No. 95-0642).

101. **Lawrence RC et al.** Estimates of the prevalence of arthritis and selected musculoskeletal disorders in the United States. *Arthritis and rheumatism*, 1998, **41**:778–799.

102. **Abenhaim L et al.** The role of activity in the therapeutic management of back pain. Report of the international Paris Task Force on Back Pain. *Spine*, 2000, **25**(suppl. 4):1–33.

103. **Engel GL.** The need for a new medical model: a challenge for biomedicine. *Science*, 1977, **196**:129–136.

104. **Loeser JD.** Schematization of pain. In: Stanton-Hicks M, Boas R, eds. *Chronic low back pain.* New York, NY, Raven Press, 1982:145–148.

105. **Waddell G et al.** Chronic low back pain. Psychological distress and illness behaviour. *Spine*, 1984, **9**:209–213.

106. **Haldeman S.** North American Spine Society presidential address: failure of the pathology model to predict back pain. *Spine*, 1990, **15**:722–724.

107. **Andresen EM, Meyers AR.** Health-related quality of life outcomes measures. *Archives of physical medicine and rehabilitation*, 2000, **81**:S30–45.

108. **Carey TS et al.** Reporting of acute low back pain in a telephone interview. Identification of potential biases. *Spine*, 1995, **20**:787–790.

109. **Palmer KT et al.** Back pain in Britain: comparison of two prevalence surveys at an interval of 10 years. *British medical journal*, 2000, **320**:1577–1578.

110. **Jin K et al.** Risk factors for work-related low back pain in the People's Republic of China. *International journal of occupational and environmental health,* 2000, **6**:26–32.

111. **Glazer PA, Clamen LM.** Differential diagnosis and management strategies of low back pain. In: Aronoff GM, ed. *Evaluation and treatment of chronic pain*, 3rd ed. Philadelphia, PA, Williams & Wilkins, 1998:225–235.

112. **Aronoff GM, Dupey DN.** Evaluation and management of back pain: preventing disability. In: Aronoff GM, ed. *Evaluation and treatment of chronic pain*, 3rd ed. Philadelphia, PA, Williams & Wilkins, 1998:247–257.

113. **Weiser S.** Psychosocial aspects of occupational musculoskeletal disorders. In: Nordin M, Andersson GBJ, Pope M, eds. *Muscusloskeletal disorders in the workplace: principles and practice.* Philadelphia, CV Mosby, 1997:52–61.

114. **Waddell G.** *The back pain revolution.* Edinburgh, Churchill Livingstone, 1998:155–262.

115. **Spitzer WO et al.** Scientific monograph of the Quebec Task Force on Whiplash Associated Disorders: redefining "whiplash" and its management. *Spine*, 1995, **20**(suppl. 8):1–73.

116. **Orthopaedic Trauma Association.** Fracture and dislocation compendium. *Journal of orthopaedic trauma,* 1996, **10**:1–155.

117. **Muller ME et al.** *The comprehensive classification of fractures of long bones.* Berlin, Springer-Verlag, 1990:54–63.

118. **Gustilo RB, Mendoza RM, Williams DN.** Problems in the management of type III (severe) open fractures. A new classification of type open fractures. *Journal of trauma,* 1984, **24**:742–746.

119. **Tscherne H, Gotzen L.** *Fractures with soft tissue injury.* Berlin, Springer-Verlag, 1984.

120. **Association for the Advancement of Automotive Medicine, Committee on Injury Scaling.** *The Abbreviated Injury Scale — 1990 Revision (AIS-90).* Des Plaines, IL, Association for the Advancement of Automotive Medicine, 1990.

121. **MacKenzie EJ, Steinwachs DM, Shankar B.** Classifying severity of trauma based on hospital discharge diagnoses: validation of an ICD-9CM to AIS-85 conversion table. *Medical care*, 1989, **27**:412–422.

122. **Sacco WJ, MacKenzie EJ, Champion HR.** Comparison of alternative methods for assessing injury severity based on anatomic descriptors. *Journal of trauma*, 1999, **47**:441–447.

123. **Jurkovich GJ et al.** The SIP as a tool to evaluate functional outcome in trauma patients. *Journal of trauma,* 1995, **39**:625–631.

124. **Butcher JL et al.** Long-term quality of life outcomes following lower extremity fractures. *Journal of trauma*, 1996, **41**:4–9.

125. **Faergemann C, Frandsen PA, Rock ND.** Expected long-term outcome after a tibial shaft fracture. *Journal of trauma*, 1999, **46**:683–686.

126. **McCarthy M, MacKenzie EJ, Ewashko T.** Determinants of rehabilitative services following an upper extremity injury. *Journal of hand therapy*, 1998, **11**:32–38.

127. **Mock C et al.** Determinants of disability following lower extremity fracture. *Journal of trauma*, 2000, **49**:1002–1011.

128. **Wesson DE et al.** The physical, psychological and socioeconomic costs of pediatric trauma. *Journal of trauma*, 1992, **33**:252–257.

129. **MacKenzie EJ et al.** Acute hospital costs of trauma in the United States: implications for regionalized systems of care. *Journal of trauma*, 1990, **30**:1096–1103.

130. **Miller T et al.** *Databook on nonfatal injury: incidence, costs and consequences.* Washington, DC, Urban Institute Press, 1994.

131. **MacKenzie EJ et al.** Return to work following injury: the role of economic, social, and job-related factors. *American journal of public health*, 1998, **88**:1630–1637.

132. **Holbrook TL et al.** Outcome after major trauma: 12-month and 18-month follow-up results from the Trauma Recovery Project. *Journal of trauma*, 1999, **46**:765–773.

133. **Ponzer S et al.** Psychosocial support in rehabilitation after orthopaedic injuries. *Journal of trauma*, 2000, **48**:273–279.

134. **Rice D.** The economic burden of musculoskeletal conditions, 1995. In: Praemer A, Furner S, Rice D. *Musculoskeletal conditions in the United States.* Rosemont, IL, American Academy of Orthopaedic Surgeons, 1999:27–33.

135. **Praemer A, Furner S, Rice D.** *Musculoskeletal conditions in the United States.* Rosemont, IL, American Academy of Orthopaedic Surgeons, 1999.

136. **Yelin E, Callahan LF, National Arthritis Data Work Group.** The economic cost and social and psychological impact of musculoskeletal conditions. *Arthritis and rheumatism,* 1995, **38**:1351–1362.

137. **Yelin E, Wanke L.** An assessment of the annual and long-term costs of rheumatoid arthritis. *Arthritis and rheumatism*, 1999, **42**:1209–1218.

138. **Salvarani C et al.** HLA-DRB1 alleles associated with rheumatoid arthritis in northern Italy: correlation with disease severity. *British journal of rheumatology*, 1998, **37**:165–169.

139. **Kvalvik AG, Jones MA, Symmons DPM.** Mortality in a cohort of Norwegian patients with rheumatoid arthritis followed from 1977 to 1992. *Scandinavian journal of rheumatology*, 2000, **29**:29–37.

140. **Pugner KM et al.** The costs of rheumatoid arthritis: an international long-term view. *Seminars in arthritis and rheumatism*, 2000, **29**:305–320.

141. **Australian Institute of Health and Welfare.** *Australian hospital statistics. 1997–98.* Canberra, Australian Institute of Health and Welfare, 1999 (AIHW Catalogue No. HSE 6. Health Services Series).

142. **Cummings S et al.** Risk factors for hip fracture in white women. *New England journal of medicine*, 1995, **332**:767–773.

143. **Burger H et al.** Added value of bone mineral density in hip fracture risk scores. *Bone*, 1999, **25**:369–374.

144. **Klotzbücher CM et al.** Patients with prior fractures have an increased risk of future fractures: a summary of the literature and statistical synthesis. *Journal of bone and mineral research*, 2000, **15**:721–739.

145. **van Staa TP et al.** Oral corticosteroids and fracture risk: relationship to daily and cumulative doses. *Rheumatology (Oxford)*, 2000, **39**:1383–1389.

146. **Ahmed AI et al.** Screening for osteopenia and osteoporosis: do the accepted normal ranges lead to osteoporosis? *Osteoporosis international*, 1997, **7**:432–438.

147. **Lips P, Ooms ME.** Non-pharmacological interventions. *Baillière's clinical endocrinology and metabolism*, 2000, **14**:265–277.

148. **Johnell O, Gullberg B, Kanis JA.** The hospital burden of vertebral fracture in Europe: a study of national register sources. *Osteoporosis international*, 1997, **7**:138–144.

149. **Jonsson B et al.** Effect and offset of effect of treatments for hip fracture on health outcomes. *Osteoporosis international*, 1999, **10**:193–199.

150. **Torgerson DJ, Reid DM.** The economics of osteoporosis and its prevention. A review. *Pharmacoeconomics*, 1997, **11**:126–138.

151. **Bovenzi M, Hulshof C.** An updated review of epidemiology studies on the relationship between exposure to whole-body vibration and low back pain (1986–1997). *International archives of occupational and environmental health*, 1999, **72**:351–365.

152. **Frymoyer JW et al.** Risk factors in low-back pain. *Journal of bone and joint surgery*, 1983, **65**:213–218.

153. **Hoogendoorn W et al.** Physical workload during work and leisure time as risk factors for back pain. *Scandinavian journal work and environmental health*, 1999, **25**:387–403.

154. **Nordin M, Andersson GBJ, Pope MH, eds.** *Musculoskeletal disorders in the workplace. Principles and practice.* Philadelphia, PA, CV Mosby, 1997.

155. **Svensson HO, Andersson GB.** Low back pain in 40- to 47-year-old men: work history and work environment factors. *Spine*, 1983, **8**:272–276.

156. **Bovim G, Schrader H, Bogduk N.** Neck pain in the general population. *Spine*, 1994, **19**:1307–1309.

157. **Heliovarra M.** Occupation and risk of herniated lumbar intervertebral disc or sciatica leading to hospitalization. *Journal of chronic disease*, 1987, **40**:259–264.

158. **Bostman OM.** Body mass index and height in patients requiring surgery for intervertebral disc herniation. *Spine*, 1993, **18**:548–552.

159. **Deyo RA, Bass E.** Lifestyle and low-back pain: the influence of smoking and obesity. *Spine*, 1989, **14**:501–506.

160. **Brown M, Tsaltas T.** Studies of the permeability of the intravertebral disc during spinal maturation. *Spine*, 1976, **1**:240–244.

161. **Colombini D et al.** Estimation of lumbar disc areas by means of anthropometric parameters. *Spine*, 1989, **4**:51–55.

162. **Nachemson A.** The effect of forward leaning on lumbar intradiscal pressure. *Acta orthopaedica Scandinavica*, 1965, **35**:314–328.

163. **Varlotta GP et al.** Familial predisposition for herniation of a lumbar disc in patients who are less than twenty-one years old. *Journal of bone and joint surgery*, 1991, **73**:124–128.

164. **Fartan H, Sullivan J.** The relation of facet orientation to intervertebral failure. *Canadian journal of surgery*, 1967, **10**:179–185.

165. **Heliovaara M et al.** Herniated lumbar disc syndrome and vertebral canals. *Spine*, 1986, **11**:433–435.

166. **Leino P, Magni G.** Depressive and distress symptoms as predictors of low back pain, neck–shoulder pain and other musculoskeletal morbidity: a 10-year follow-up of metal industry workers. *Pain*, 1993, **53**:89–94.

167. **Nagi SZ et al.** A social epidemiology of back pain in a general population. *Journal of chronic disease*, 1973, **26**:769–779.

168. **Lindgren B.** The economic impact of musculoskeletal disorders. *Acta orthopaedica Scandinavica supplementum*, 1998, **281**:58–60.

169. **Rice DP.** *Estimating the costs of illness.* Washington, DC, United States Government Printing Office, 1966 (Health Economics Series, No. 6).

170. **Jacobson L, Lindgren B.** *Vad Kostar Sjukdomarna?* [*What are the costs of illness?*] Stockholm, Socialstyrelsen [National Board of Health and Welfare], 1996.

171. **Frymoyer JW, Durett CL.** The economics of spinal disorders. In: Frymoyer JW, ed. *The adult spine: principles and practice.* Philadelphia, PA, Lippincott-Raven, 1997:143–150.

172. **Badley EM, Crotty M.** An international comparison of the estimated effect of the aging of the population on the major cause of disablement, musculoskeletal disorders. *Journal of rheumatology*, 1995, **22**:1934–1940.

173. **Bonnie RJ, Fulco CF, Liverman CT, eds.** *Reducing the burden of injury: advancing prevention and treatment.* Washington, DC, National Academy Press, 1999.

174. **Tinetti ME, Speechley M, Ginter SF.** Risk factors for falls among elderly persons living in the community. *New England journal of medicine*, 1988, **319**:1701–1707.

175. **MacKenzie EJ, Fowler CJ.** Epidemiology. In: Mattox KL, Feliciano DV, Moore EE, eds. *Trauma.* New York, NY, McGraw-Hill, 2000:21–40.

176. **Ross PD et al.** Pain and disability associated with new vertebral fractures and other spinal conditions. *Journal of clinical epidemiology*, 1994, **47**:231–239.

177. **Gabriel SE et al.** Health related quality of life in the economic evaluations for osteoporosis: whose values should we use? *Medical decision making*, 1999, **19**:141–148.

178. **National Osteoporosis Foundation.** Osteoporosis: a review of the evidence for prevention, diagnosis and treatment and cost-effectiveness analysis. *Osteoporosis international*, 1998, **8**:1–88.

179. **Salkeld G et al.** Quality of life related to fear of falling and hip fracture in older women: a time trade off study. *British medical journal*, 2000, **320**:341–346.

180. **Cohen ME, Marino JR.** The tools of disability outcomes research functional status measures. *Archives of physical medicine and rehabilitation*, 2000, **81**(suppl. 2):S21–S29.

181. **Mahoney FI, Barthel DW.** Functional evaluation: the Barthel Index. *Maryland State medical journal,* 1965, **14**:61–65.

182. **Hamilton BB et al.** A uniform national data system for medical rehabilitation. In: Fuhrer MJ, ed. *Rehabilitation outcomes: analysis and measurement.* Baltimore, MD, Paula H Brookes, 1987.

183. **Bergner M et al.** The SIP: development and final revision of a health status measure. *Medical care,* 1981, **9**:787–805.

184. **Ware JE, Sherbourne CD.** The MOS 36-item Short-Form Health Survey (SF-36). I. Conceptual framework and item selection. *Medical care,* 1992, **30**:473–483.

185. **Ware JE, Kosinski M, Keller SD.** A 12-item Short-Form Health Survey: construction of scales and preliminary tests of reliability and validity. *Medical care*, 1996, **3**:220–233.

186. **Landgraf JM, Abetz LN, Ware JE.** *The CHQ User's Manual.* Boston, MA, Health Institute, New England Medical Center, 1996.

187. **Kaplan RM, Bush JW.** Health-related quality of life measurement for evaluation research and policy analysis. *Health psychology*, 1982, **1**:61–80.

188. **Feeny D et al.** Multi-attribute health status classification systems: the Health Utilities Index. *Pharmacoeconomics*, 1995, **7**:490–502.

189. **EuroQol Group.** EuroQol: a new facility for the measurement of health-related quality of life. *Health policy*, 1990, **16**:199–208.

190. **MacKenzie EJ et al.** The development of the Functional Capacity Index. *Journal of trauma*, 1996, **41**:799–807.

191. **Martin DP et al.** Development of a musculoskeletal extremity health status instrument: the Musculoskeletal Function Assessment instrument. *Journal of orthopedic research,* 1996, **l4**:113–181.

192. **Spilker B.** *Quality of life and pharmacoeconomics in clinical trials*, 2nd ed. Philadelphia, PA, Lippincott-Raven, 1996.

Annex

Estimates of incidence or prevalence of key musculoskeletal disorders considered for each WHO region

To aid in cause of death analyses, burden of disease analyses and comparative risk assessment, the 191 Member States of WHO have been divided into the six WHO regions (African Region, Region of the Americas, South-East Asia Region, European Region, Eastern Mediterranean Region, and the Western Pacific Region). These are further divided into mortality strata on thc basis of thcir lcvcls of child mortality under 5 years of age and mortality among men aged 15–59 years.

The mortality strata are defined as follows:

A: very low child, very low adult
B: low child, low adult
C: low child, high adult
D: high child, high adult
E: high child, very high adult.

Estimates of incidence and prevalence for rheumatoid arthritis, osteoarthritis (hip, knee), osteoporosis (fracture), spinal disorders and limb trauma are summarized below in Tables 1–118. For additional information on the methodology being employed here in estimating burden of disease, see Section 2 of the main report.

Rheumatoid arthritis

Data for the age group 0–14 years relate to juvenile idiopathic arthritis, the preferred definition being either the American Rheumatism Association (ARA) criteria for juvenile rheumatoid arthritis or the EULAR criteria for juvenile chronic arthritis. Data for adults relate to rheumatoid arthritis, the preferred definition being either the 1987 ACR criteria (*1*) or the 1958 ARA criteria (*2*). The 1958 criteria assign a certainty level depending upon the number of positive criteria present: 3 or 4 is probable, 5 or 6 is definite, and 7 or 8 is classical. Cases classified as definite or classical are more likely indicative of rheumatoid arthritis.

African Region — D

Table 1
Prevalence of rheumatoid arthritis[a] per 100 000 population in West Africa

	Age groups (years)					
	5–14	15–24	25–34	35–44	45–54	≥55
Males	—	—	—	3333	1538	7246
Females	—	—	1042	2062	2740	5000

[a] Includes probable plus definite cases.
Source: reference *3*.

African Region — E

Table 2
Prevalence of rheumatoid arthritis[a] per 100 000 population[b] in South Africa

	Age groups (years)						
	15–24	25–34	35–44	45–54	55–64	65–74	≥75
Males	—	—	2857	2740	3846	4286	8000
Females	—	—	—	2564	3704	6173	6061

[a] Includes probable plus definite cases.
[b] Combined data from three studies.
Source: references *4–6*.

Region of the Americas — A

Table 3
Prevalence of rheumatoid arthritis per 100 000 population in the USA

	Age groups (years)[a]						
	0–4	5–14	35–44	45–59	60–69	70–79	≥80
Males	4[b]	39	97	429	1264	1793	1619
Females	33	167	300	1203	2601	2087	2476

[a] There are no data for the age band 15–34 years.
[b] Estimated from the data set.
Source: references *7* and *8* and S.E. Gabriel, unpublished data, 2002.

Region of the Americas — B

Table 4
Prevalence of rheumatoid arthritis per 100 000 population in Jamaica

	Age groups (years)		
	35–44	45–54	55–64
Males	—	—	2841
Females	544	1205	1630

Source: reference *9*.

Region of the Americas — D

The Scientific Group did not find appropriate data sets for Region of the Americas — D and therefore suggested using data from Region of the Americas — B.

South-East Asia Region — B

Table 5

Prevalence of rheumatoid arthritis per 100 000 population in Indonesia

	Age groups (years)					
	15–24	25–34	35–44	45–54	55–64	≥65
Males	—	—	—	—	422	1220
Females	—	279	—	—	752	2581

Source: reference *10*.

South-East Asia Region — D

Tablo 6

Prevalence of rheumatoid arthritis per 100 000 population in India

	Age groups (years)				
	15–29	30–44	45–59	60–74	≥75
Males	—	479	—	1136	—
Females	113	1639	1775	1914	3846

Source: A. Chopra, unpublished data from Bhigwan COPCORD Study (India).

European Region — A

Table 7

Prevalence of rheumatoid arthritis per 100 000 population in Norway (adults) and Sweden (children)

	Age groups (years)[a]					
	0–16	20–39	40–49	50–59	60–69	70–79
Males	64	45	93	245	487	715
Females	108	150	426	925	1533	1745

[a] There are no data for the age band 17–19 years.
Source: references *11* (adults) and *12* (children).

European Region — B

Table 8

Prevalence of rheumatoid arthritis per 100 000 population in Bulgaria

	Age groups (years)					
	15–24	25–34	35–44	45–54	55–64	≥65
Males	—	614	328	606	273[a]	360[a]
Females	—	800	2000	2500	1250	435

[a] Estimated from the data set.
Source: reference *13*.

European Region — C

The Scientific Group did not identify appropriate data sets from European Region — C and therefore suggested using data from European Region — B.

Eastern Mediterranean Region — B

Table 9

Prevalence of rheumatoid arthritis per 100 000 population in Kuwait

	Age groups (years)						
	0–16	15–24	25–34	35–44	45–54	55–64	≥65
Males	19	—	—	—	—	—	—
Females	25	—	—	—	—	—	—

Source: reference *14*.

Eastern Mediterranean Region — D

Table 10

Prevalence of rheumatoid arthritis per 100 000 population in Iraq

	Age groups (years)						
	0–4	5–15	16–24	25–34	45–54	55–64	≥65
Males	—	—	22	218	550	1204	1518
Females	—	—	78	742	1870	4096	5162

Source: reference *15*.

Western Pacific Region — A

The Scientific Group did not identify appropriate data sets from Western Pacific Region — A and therefore suggested using data from Region of the Americas — A.

Western Pacific Region — B

Table 11
Prevalence of rheumatoid arthritis per 100 000 population in China

	Age groups (years)						
	18–24	25–34	35–44	45–54	55–64	65–74	75–79
Males	0	145	216	1066	260	372	1299
Females	0	145	237	1459	1136	888	1770

Source: references *16* and *17*.

Osteoarthritis of the hip

The preferred definition is that of symptoms plus radiographic changes. Radiographic changes may be graded 0–4 based on the methodology developed by Kellgren & Lawrence with grade 4 being the most severe (*18*). However, because most studies consider radiographic changes alone, the Scientific Group has preferentially selected these studies in order to permit comparison between regions. The Scientific Group has also been obliged to present the data for very wide age groups, since most studies are not sufficiently large to permit narrower ones. Where possible, data for Kellgren & Lawrence grades 2–4 and 3–4 from the same study are presented.

African Region — D

The Scientific Group did not identify appropriate data sets from African Region — D and therefore suggested using data from African Region — E.

African Region — E

Table 12
Prevalence of osteoarthritis of the hip per 100 000 population in South Africa

	Age band (years)
	≥55
Males	3278
Females	2899

Source: reference *19*.

Region of the Americas — A

Table 13
Prevalence of osteoarthritis of the hip[a] per 100 000 population in the USA

	Age groups (years)				
	25–34	35–44	45–54	55–64	65–74
Males	400	100	700	2600	4600
Females	NA	NA	800[b]	2800	2700

NA: data not available for females under 45 years.
[a] Cases based on Kellgren and Lawrence grades 2–4.
[b] Ages 50–54 years for females.
Source: reference *20.*

Table 14
Prevalence of osteoarthritis of the hip[a] per 100 000 population in the USA

	Age groups (years)				
	25–34	35–44	45–54	55–64	65–74
Males	200	—	100	700	1300
Females	NA	NA	100[b]	1600	1200

NA: data not available for females under 45 years.
[a] Cases based on Kellgren & Lawrence grades 3–4.
[b] Ages 50–54 years for females.
Source: reference *20.*

Region of the Americas — B

Table 15
Prevalence of osteoarthritis of the hip[a] per 100 000 population in Jamaica

	Age band (years)
	55–64
Males	1000
Females	4000

[a] Cases based on Kellgren & Lawrence grades 2–4.
Source: reference *21.*

Region of the Americas — D

The Scientific Group did not identify appropriate data sets from Region of the Americas — D and therefore suggested using data from African Region — E.

South-East Asia Region — B

The Scientific Group did not identify appropriate data sets from South-East Asia Region — B and therefore suggested using data from Western Pacific Region — B.

South-East Asia Region — D

The Scientific Group did not identify appropriate data sets from South-East Asia Region — D and therefore suggested using data from Western Pacific Region — B.

European Region — A

Table 16

Prevalence of osteoarthritis of the hip[a] per 100000 population in Sweden

	Age groups (years)				
	40–49	50–59	60–69	70–79	≥80
Males	—	237	1250	4450	4142
Females	—	806	1426	3984	6201

[a] Cases based on radiographically assessed joint space of less than 4 mm if aged under 70 years, and less than 3 mm if aged 70 years or over.

Source: reference *22*.

European Region — B

Table 17

Prevalence of osteoarthritis of the hip[a] per 100000 population in Bulgaria[b]

	Age groups (years)				
	25–34	35–44	45–54	55–64	≥65
Males	613	327	—	1515	2121
Females	200	444	1346	625	1304

[a] Case definition not specified.

[b] Phase I of this study involved a random population sample from Sofia. These results are from phase II, which included only the positive responders with rheumatic or cardiovascular complaints (27% of the sample surveyed).

Source: reference *23*.

European Region — D

The Scientific Group did not identify appropriate data sets from European Region — D and therefore suggested using data from European Region — B.

Eastern Mediterranean Region — B

The Scientific Group did not identify appropriate data sets from Eastern Mediterranean Region — B and therefore suggested using the following data set from Israel.

Table 18

Prevalence of osteoarthritis of the hip[a] per 100 000 population in Israel

	Age groups (years)			
	45–54	55–64	65–74	75–84
Males	0	2439	9302	2913
Females	0	3947	5682	6098

[a] Cases based on Kellgren & Lawrence grades 3–4.
Source: reference *24*.

Eastern Mediterranean Region — D

The Scientific Group did not identify appropriate data sets from Eastern Mediterranean Region — D and therefore suggested using data from Israel as for Eastern Mediterranean Region — B.

Western Pacific Region — A

The Scientific Group identified only one appropriate data set from Western Pacific Region — A. The Scientific Group suggested using data from Region of the Americas — A for Australia and New Zealand, and using the following data for Japan.

Table 19

Prevalence of osteoarthritis of the hip[a] per 100 000 population in Japan

	Age groups (years)				
	35–44	45–54	55–64	65–74	≥75
Males	1075	961	4597	6897	10349
Females	5000	6977	5128	11667	26471

[a] Cases based on Kellgren & Lawrence grades 2–4.
Source: reference *25*.

Table 20

Prevalence of osteoarthritis of the hip[a] per 100 000 population in Japan

	Age groups (years)			
	55–64	65–74	75–84	≥85
Males	—	—	3846	—
Females	—	—	9375	50000

[a] Cases based on Kellgren & Lawrence grades 3–4.
Source: reference *25*.

Western Pacific Region — B

Table 21

Prevalence of osteoarthritis of the hip[a] per 100 000 population in Hong Kong SAR, China

	Age groups (years)			
	55–64	65–74	75–84	≥85
Males	650	2700	—	—
Females	—	1250	—	33 300

[a] Cases based on Kellgren & Lawrence grades 3–4.
Source: reference *26*.

Osteoarthritis of the knee

The preferred definition is that of symptoms plus radiographic changes. Most studies, however, consider either radiographic changes alone or symptoms alone. As an approximate guide, 50% of people with X-ray changes of Kellgren & Lawrence grades 2–4 have pain, and vice versa, the prevalence of pain being higher in persons with grades 3–4. Where possible the Scientific Group presents data for both grades 2–4 and 3–4 from the same study.

African Region — D

The Scientific Group did not identify appropriate data sets from African Region — D and therefore suggested using data from African Region — E.

African Region — E

Table 22

Prevalence of osteoarthritis of the knee[a] per 100 000 population in South Africa

	Age band (years)
	≥35
Males	20 238
Females	38 208

[a] Cases based on clinical assessment
Source: reference *27*.

Region of the Americas — A

Table 23
Prevalence of osteoarthritis of the knee[a] per 100 000 population in the USA

	Age groups (years)					
	25–34	35–44	45–54	55–64	65–74	≥75
Males	—	1750	2270	4040	8380	30500
Females	100	1440	3560	7240	17970	41800

[a] Cases based on Kellgren & Lawrence grades 2–4.
Source: references *28* and *29*.

Table 24
Prevalence of osteoarthritis of the knee[a] per 100 000 population in the USA

	Age groups (years)					
	25–34	35–44	45–54	55–64	65–74	≥75
Males	—	100	200	1000	1500	—
Females	—	500	500	900	6600	—

[a] Cases based on Kellgren & Lawrence grades 3–4.
Source: reference *20*.

Region of the Americas — B

Table 25
Prevalence of osteoarthritis of the knee[a] per 100 000 population in Jamaica

	Age band (years)
	35–64
Males	19000
Females	28000

[a] Cases based on Kellgren & Lawrence grades 2–4.
Source: reference *21*.

Table 26
Prevalence of osteoarthritis of the knee[a] per 100 000 population in Jamaica

	Age band (years)
	35–64
Males	3000
Females	7000

[a] Cases based on Kellgren & Lawrence grades 3–4.
Source: reference *21*.

Region of the Americas — D

The Scientific Group did not identify appropriate data sets from Region of the Americas — D and therefore suggested using data from Region of the Americas — B.

South-East Asia Region — B

The Scientific Group did not identify appropriate data sets from South-East Asia Region — B and therefore suggested using data from South-East Asia Region — D.

South-East Asia Region — D

Table 27

Prevalence of osteoarthritis of the knee[a] per 100 000 population in India

	Age groups (years)						
	15–24	25–34	35–44	45–59	60–69	70–79	≥80
Males	—	—	—	4644	15 385	20 000	6 250
Females	—	—	2247	6587	14 371	19 608	14 286

[a] Cases based on clinical ACR criteria (*17*).
Source: A. Chopra, unpublished data from Bhigwan COPCORD Study (India).

European Region — A

Table 28

Prevalence of osteoarthritis of the knee[a] per 100 000 population in the Netherlands

	Age groups (years)					
	25–34	35–44	45–54	55–64	65–74	≥75
Males	—	—	9 300	16 800	20 900	22 100
Females	—	—	13 900	18 500	35 200	44 100

[a] Cases based on Kellgren & Lawrence grades 2–4.
Source: reference *30*.

Table 29

Prevalence of osteoarthritis of the knee[a] per 100 000 population in Spain

	Age groups (years)						
	20–29	30–39	40–49	50–59	60–69	70–79	≥80
Males	—	962	2381	5 479	18 121	16 667	14 286
Females	885	433	4433	13 333	37 195	44 095	25 532

[a] Cases based on clinical, ACR criteria (*31*).
Source: reference *32* and L Carmona, unpublished data, 1999.

European Region — B

Table 30
Prevalence of osteoarthritis of the knee[a] per 100 000 population in Bulgaria[b]

	Age groups (years)					
	15–24	25–34	35–44	45–54	55–64	≥65
Males	1200	3067	3607	6970	10 000	9600
Females	196	1600	4667	9615	11 250	9565

[a] Cases based on unspecified radiographic findings.
[b] Phase I of this study involved a random population sample from Sofia. These results are from phase II, which included only the positive responders with rheumatic or cardiovascular complaints (27% of the sample surveyed).
Source: reference *23*.

European Region — C

The Scientific Group did not identify appropriate data sets from European Region — C and therefore suggested using data from European Region — B.

Eastern Mediterranean Region — B

The Scientific Group did not identify appropriate data sets from Eastern Mediterranean Region — B and therefore suggested using data from Eastern Mediterranean Region — D.

Eastern Mediterranean Region — D

Table 31
Prevalence of osteoarthritis of the knee[a] per 100 000 population in Pakistan

	Age groups (years)					
	15–24	25–34	35–44	45–54	55–64	≥65
Males	—	—	—	1014	3086	4511
Females	—	—	1136	4615	9302	6383

[a] Cases based on clinical symptoms plus varus deformity; the data presented are for poor and affluent populations combined.
Source: reference *33*.

Western Pacific Region — A

The Scientific Group identified only one appropriate data set from Western Pacific Region — A and therefore suggested using data from Region of the Americas — A for Australia and New Zealand, and using the following data for Japan.

Table 32
Prevalence of osteoarthritis of the knee[a] per 100 000 population in Japan

	Age band (years)
	40–65
Males	26 100
Females	12 000

[a] Cases based on joint space narrowing assessed through radiographs.
Source: reference *34*.

Western Pacific Region — B

Table 33
Prevalence of osteoarthritis of the knee[a] per 100 000 population in Hong Kong SAR, China

	Age groups (years)			
	55–64	65–74	75–84	≥85
Males	2000	9000	6000	67 000
Females	7000	16 000	30 000	—

[a] Cases based on Kellgren & Lawrence grades 3–4.
Source: reference *28*.

Osteoporosis: incidence of fractured proximal femur

African Region — D

Table 34
Incidence of proximal femur fracture per 100 000 population in Nigeria

	Age groups (years)			
	50–54	55–64	65–74	≥75
Males	—	2	2	8
Females	—	2	2	—

Source: reference *35*.

African Region — E

Table 35
Incidence of proximal femur fracture per 100 000 population in South Africa

	Age groups (years)										
	30–34	35–39	40–44	45–49	50–54	55–59	60–64	65–69	70–74	75–79	≥80
Males	3	2	3	3	6	10	14	27	8	—	116
Females	—	1	3	1	4	12	17	12	16	50	80

Source: reference *36*.

Region of the Americas — A

Table 36
Incidence of proximal femur fracture per 100 000 population in the USA

	Age groups (years)										
	35–39	40–44	45–49	50–54	55–59	60–64	65–69	70–74	75–79	80–84	≥85
Males	8	19	0	40	32	81	189	160	534	597	1501
Females	7	18	32	66	83	165	221	275	861	1838	2488

Source: reference *37*.

Region of the Americas — B

Table 37
Incidence of proximal femur fracture per 100 000 population in Brazil

	Age groups (years)							
	20–29	30–39	40–49	50–59	60–69	70–79	80–89	≥90
Males	19	9	21	26	106	159	618	1144
Females	3	0	13	35	84	531	1263	2252

Source: reference *38*.

Region of the Americas — D

Table 38
Incidence of proximal femur fracture per 100 000 population in Chile

	Age groups (years)					
	50–59	60–64	65–69	70–74	75–79	≥80
Males	29	9	17	28	48	58
Females	13	14	30	26	109	204

Source: reference *39*.

South-East Asia Region — B

Table 39
Incidence of proximal femur fracture per 100 000 population in Thailand

	Age groups (years)					
	50–54	55–59	60–64	65–69	70–74	≥75
Males	27	36	35	77	144	390
Females	10	59	89	148	361	704

Source: reference *40*.

South-East Asia Region — D

Table 40
Incidence of proximal femur fracture per 100 000 population in the Republic of Korea

	Age groups (years)			
	50–59	60–69	70–79	≥80
Males	21	35	67	214
Females	9	22	66	130

Source: reference *41*.

European Region — A

Table 41
Incidence of proximal femur fracture per 100 000 population in the United Kingdom

	Age groups (years)							
	50–54	55–59	60–64	65–69	70–74	75–79	80–84	≥85
Males	13	29	57	108	196	340	571	1470
Females	18	43	93	191	373	695	1250	3620

Source: reference *42*.

European Region — B

Table 42
Incidence of proximal femur fracture per 100 000 population in rural areas of Turkey

	Age groups (years)								
	50–54	55–59	60–64	65–69	70–74	75–79	80–84	85–89	≥90
Males	26	23	56	98	79	73	370	300	—
Females	2	17	31	50	34	27	35	100	—

Source: reference *43*.

European Region — C

Table 43
Incidence of proximal femur fracture per 100 000 population in Budapest, Hungary

	Age groups (years)												
	20–29	30–39	40–49	50–54	55–59	60–64	65–69	70–74	75–79	80–84	85–89	90–95	≥95
Males	0	6	42	54	72	129	158	240	280	728	1499	1873	—
Females	3	6	25	39	46	84	193	288	565	1101	1653	2217	—

Source: reference *44*.

Eastern Mediterranean Region — B

Table 44
Incidence of proximal femur fracture per 100 000 population in Kuwait

	Age groups (years)							
	10–19	20–29	30–39	40–49	50–59	60–69	70–79	≥80
Males	5	5	7	16	50	96	349	1113
Females	2	2	2	1	28	124	458	1189

Source: reference *45*.

Eastern Mediterranean Region — D

The Scientific Group did not identify appropriate data sets for this region and therefore suggested using data from the Republic of Korea, which is in the same mortality band. The alternative would be to use data from Kuwait, which is geographically nearer but much more affluent.

Western Pacific Region — A

Table 45
Incidence of proximal femur fracture per 100 000 population in Australia

	Age groups (years)											
	35–39	40–44	45–49	50–54	55–59	60–64	65–69	70–74	75–79	80–84	85–89	≥90
Males	12	—	39	52	103	92	114	424	772	856	3852	5263
Females	—	12	—	17	81	65	334	633	1599	2769	6687	7496

Source: reference *46*.

Western Pacific Region — B

Table 46
Incidence of proximal femur fracture per 100 000 population in Beijing, China

	Age groups (years)											
	20–29	30–39	40–49	50–54	55–59	60–64	65–69	70–74	75–79	80–84	85–89	≥90
Males	2	6	11	19	33	84	88	133	161	282	328	445
Females	1	3	8	18	32	56	91	164	141	224	219	401

Source: reference *44*.

Spinal disorders: lifetime prevalence of adolescent idiopathic scoliosis

World

Table 47

Lifetime prevalence of adolescent idiopathic scoliosis[a] per 100 000 population

	Age band (years)
	13–16
Males	2000–3000
Females	2000–3000

[a] Based on data from Israel, Italy, Poland, South Africa, the United Kingdom and the USA, 1957–1988, diagnosed by the presence of at least 10 degrees of deviation by the Cobb method (*47*).

Source: reference *48*.

Spinal disorders: nonspecific spinal disorders (back pain)

The preferred definition of back pain was pain lasting at least one week and associated with some disability. There are surprisingly few studies of back pain (using any definition) which provide an age-specific and sex-specific prevalence. The studies in this annex are grouped by point, monthly, annual and lifetime prevalence. These are subdivided into those reporting the experience of back pain and those reporting back pain lasting at least one week. None of the studies presented here uses the same definition. Consequently, it is not possible to make many direct comparisons. The Scientific Group suggested using data from areas of similar mortality where this is feasible, rather than from adjacent areas.

Point prevalence of experiencing back pain

African Region — E

Table 48

Point prevalence of experiencing back pain per 100 000 population in Kenya, 1982–1987

	Age group (years)
	11–75
Males	7 400
Females	12 600

Source: reference *49*.

South-East Asia Region — B

Table 49

Point prevalence of experiencing back pain[a] per 100 000 population in rural Indonesia, 1994

	Age groups (years)					
	15–24	25–34	35–44	45–54	55–64	≥65
Males	3971	17969	34626	22713	34426	54962
Females	17979	17778	18204	17994	21782	32727

[a] Paralumbar myalgia.
Source: reference *50* and J. Darmawan, personal communication, 1999.

European Region — A

Table 50

Point prevalence of experiencing back pain[a] per 100 000 population in Denmark, 1998

	Age group (years)
	13–16
Males	4300
Females	6100

[a] Low back pain.
Source: reference *51*.

Table 51

Point prevalence of experiencing back pain per 100 000 population in Sweden, 1996

	Age groups (years)			
	20–29	30–39	40–49	50–59
Males	24000	23000	30000	28000
Females	25000	31000	32000	33000

Source: reference *52*.

Table 52

Point prevalence of experiencing back pain per 100 000 population in the United Kingdom, 1998

	Age groups (years)				
	16–24	25–44	45–54	55–64	≥65
Males	3000	12000	18000	17000	17000
Females	10000	10000	16000	20000	22000

Source: reference *53*.

Eastern Mediterranean Region — B

Table 53

Point prevalence of experiencing back pain[a] per 100 000 population in Lebanon, 1984

	Age group (years)
	Unknown
Males	2500
Females	5300

[a] Low back pain.
Source: reference *54*.

Western Pacific Region — A

Table 54

Point prevalence of experiencing back pain[a] per 100 000 population in Japan, 1992

	Age groups (years)				
	<20	20–29	30–39	40–49	50–59
Males	18 300	20 000	25 500	36 500	35 300
Females	21 100	18 100	20 000	29 300	29 400

[a] Low back pain.
Source: reference *55*.

Table 55

Point prevalence of experiencing back pain per 100 000 population in New Zealand, 1987–1988

	Age group (years)
	≥15
Males	17 500
Females	17 500

Source: reference *56*.

Table 56

Point prevalence of experiencing back pain per 100 000 population in New Zealand, 1992

	Age groups (years)		
	<35	35–45	>45
Males	9100	13 600	13 100
Females	9800	12 100	13 800

Source: reference *57*.

Western Pacific Region — B

Table 57

Point prevalence of experiencing back pain[a] per 100 000 population in the Philippines, 1983

	Age groups (years)			
	5–14	15–44	45–64	≥65
Males	—	5400	12 000	20 700
Females	500	3800	19 600	11 100

[a] Lumbar pain.
Source: reference *58*.

Point prevalence of severe or frequent pain, or pain lasting more than seven days

African Region — E

Table 58

Point prevalence of severe back[a] pain per 100 000 population in Lesotho, 1993

	Age group (years)
	15–44
Males	—
Females	10 120

[a] Low back pain.
Source: reference *59*.

Region of the Americas — A

Table 59

Point prevalence of severe back pain[a] per 100 000 population in the USA, 1996

	Age groups (years)									
	0–4	5–14	15–24	25–34	35–44	45–54	55–64	65–74	75–84	≥85
Males	—	—	1210	2010	5210	9250	8990	9520	8010	9400
Females	—	—	1520	2350	3180	10 220	11 690	10 070	10 740	4890

[a] Self-reported chronic, disabling low back pain.
Source: reference *60*.

European Region — A

Table 60

Point prevalence of severe back pain[a] per 100 000 population in Denmark, 1995

	Age groups (years)	
	12–14	15–41
Males	6000	19 000
Females	6000	19 000

[a] Pain lasting more than seven days.
Source: reference *61*.

Table 61

Point prevalence of severe back pain[a] per 100 000 population in Sweden, 1960–1971

	Age band (years)
	40–47
Males	7800
Females	—

[a] Low back pain in males in the city of Goteborg.
Source: reference *62*.

Western Pacific Region — A

Table 62

Point prevalence of severe back pain[a] per 100 000 population in New Zealand, 1987–1988

	Age band (years)
	15+
Males	8500
Females	8500

[a] Pain lasting more than seven days.
Source: reference *56*.

Month prevalence of experiencing back pain

Region of the Americas — B

Table 63

Month prevalence of experiencing back pain[a] per 100 000 population in Brazil, 1999

	Age band (years)
	≥16
Males	31 300
Females	31 300

[a] Low back pain.
Source: reference *63*.

European Region — A

Table 64

Month prevalence of experiencing back pain per 100 000 population in Sweden, 1989–1991

	Age groups (years)					
	38–39	40–44	45–49	50–54	55–59	60–64
Males	—	—	—	—	—	—
Females	29 800	36 900	30 900	34 100	37 000	41 600

Source: reference *64*.

Month prevalence of severe or frequent pain, or pain lasting more than seven days

European Region — A

Table 65
Month prevalence of severe back pain[a] per 100 000 population in Sweden, 1989–1991

	Age groups (years)					
	38–39	40–44	45–49	50–54	55–59	60–64
Males	—	—	—	—	—	—
Females	8080	9850	5560	11 940	10 030	16 850

[a] Severe or disabling pain.
Source: reference *64*.

Western Pacific Region — A

Table 66
Month prevalence of severe back pain[a] per 100 000 population in Australia, 1995

	Age groups (years)								
	0–4	5–14	15–24	25–34	35–44	45–54	55–64	65–74	≥75
Males	—	100	900	1220	2540	3230	3060	2020	4210
Females	—	70	530	1740	1830	2630	2680	2070	3230

[a] Disabling back pain in the past two weeks.
Source: reference *65*.

Annual prevalence of experiencing back pain

African Region — E

Table 67
Annual prevalence of back pain[a] per 100 000 population in South Africa, 1992

	Age band (years)
	15–44
Males	20 000
Females	20 000

[a] Workers with low back pain since starting their current jobs.
Source: reference *66*.

Region of the Americas — A

Table 68

Annual prevalence of back pain[a] per 100 000 population in Canada, 1985–1995

	Age groups (years)	
	60–69	70–79
Males	21 000	25 000
Females	26 000	39 000

[a] Low back pain.
Source: reference *67*.

Table 69

Annual prevalence of back pain[a] per 100 000 population in the USA, 1985

	Age band (years)
	18–70
Males	56 000
Females	56 000

[a] Back pain lasting one or more days.
Source: reference *68*.

Table 70

Annual prevalence of back pain[a] per 100 000 population in the USA, 1992–1993

	Age groups (years)	
	68–80	81–100
Males	43 000	38 000
Females	53 000	51 000

[a] Low back pain.
Source: reference *69*.

South-East Asia Region — D

Table 71

Annual prevalence of back pain[a] per 100 000 population in India, 1988

	Age band (years)
	15–44
Males	61 000
Females	—

[a] Low back pain.
Source: reference *70*.

Table 72
Annual prevalence of back pain per 100 000 population in Nepal, 1982

	Age band (years)
	≥15
Males	17 300
Females	18 400

Source: reference *71*.

European Region — A

Table 73
Annual prevalence of back pain[a] per 100 000 population in Denmark, 1998

	Age band (years)
	13–16
Males	49 300
Females	52 100

[a] Low back pain.
Source: reference *51*.

Table 74
Annual prevalence of back pain per 100 000 population in Sweden, 1996

	Age groups (years)			
	20–29	30–39	40–49	50–59
Males	49 000	54 000	64 000	59 000
Females	54 000	55 000	52 000	59 000

Source: reference *52*.

Table 75
Annual prevalence of back pain per 100 000 population in Sweden, 1994

	Age groups (years)		
	77–79	80–84	≥85
Males	39 300	33 300	35 600
Females	53 300	45 100	44 400

Source: reference *72*.

Table 76
Annual prevalence of back pain per 100 000 population in the United Kingdom, 1997–1998

	Age groups (years)			
	20–29	30–39	40–49	50–59
Males	46 500	52 400	56 400	56 600
Females	46 500	52 400	56 400	56 600

Source: reference *73*.

Table 77

Annual prevalence of back pain per 100 000 population in the United Kingdom, 1987–1988

	Age groups (years)			
	20–29	30–39	40–49	50–59
Males	34 900	38 100	37 000	40 200
Females	34 900	38 100	37 000	40 200

Source: reference *73*.

Table 78

Annual prevalence of back pain per 100 000 population in the United Kingdom, 1998

	Age groups (years)				
	16–24	25–44	45–54	55–64	≥65
Males	30 000	36 000	48 000	49 000	35 000
Females	35 000	37 000	43 000	47 000	42 000

Source: reference *53*.

Western Pacific Region — A

Table 79

Annual prevalence of back pain per 100 000 population in New Zealand, 1987–1988

	Age band (years)
	≥15
Males	63 700
Females	63 700

Source: reference *56*.

Table 80

Annual prevalence of back pain per 100 000 population in New Zealand, 1992

	Age groups (years)		
	<35	35–45	>45
Males	38 700	31 150	33 500
Females	40 700	33 500	35 500

Source: reference *57*.

Western Pacific Region — B

Table 81

Annual prevalence of back pain[a] per 100 000 population in Hong Kong SAR, China, 1990

	Age groups (years)		
	70–79	80–89	≥90
Males	22 000	24 000	36 000
Females	56 000	55 000	51 000

[a] Back pain: lumbar or thoracic (55–64% with pain report the pain as limiting activity).
Source: reference *67*.

Table 82

Annual prevalence of back pain per 100 000 population in Tokeleau, 1982

	Age groups (years)							
	15–19	20–24	25–34	35–44	45–54	55–64	65–74	≥75
Males	4900	12 100	11 800	22 500	21 700	24 400	12 500	18 100
Females	4400	2000	15 700	9400	14 300	21 300	22 200	14 300

Source: reference *74*.

Table 83

Annual prevalence of back pain[a] per 100 000 population in Hong Kong SAR, China, 1994

	Age groups (years)						
	<20	20–29	30–39	40–49	50–59	60–69	≥70
Males	3000	22 000	9000	4000	4000	8000	3000
Females	5000	22 000	15 000	9000	14 000	14 000	7000

[a] Low back pain.
Source: reference *36*.

Annual prevalence of back pain that is severe or frequent or lasts more than seven days

Region of the Americas — A

Table 84

Annual prevalence of severe back pain[a] per 100 000 population in the USA, 1985

	Age groups (years)			
	18–34	35–49	50–64	≥65
Males	13 240	17 290	17 630	15 650
Females	17 560	22 910	23 370	20 750

[a] Frequent back pain in the past 12 months.
Source: reference *75*.

Table 85

Annual prevalence of severe back pain[a] per 100 000 population in the USA, 1992–1993

	Age groups (years)	
	68–80	81–100
Males	18 000	13 000
Females	25 000	27 000

[a] Low back pain on most days.
Source: reference *69*.

European Region — A

Table 86

Annual prevalence of severe back pain[a] per 100 000 population in Denmark, 1998

	Age group (years)
	13–16
Males	13 100
Females	25 300

[a] Low back pain.
Source: reference *51*.

Table 87

Annual prevalence of severe back pain[a] per 100 000 population in Switzerland

	Age groups (years)				
	25–34	35–44	45–54	55–64	65–74
Males	20 200	20 300	28 300	27 900	28 500
Females	31 100	27 100	29 900	36 300	38 500

[a] Low back pain for more than seven cumulative days.
Source: reference *76*.

Table 88

Annual prevalence of severe back pain per 100 000 population in the United Kingdom, 1997–1998

	Age groups (years)			
	20–29	30–39	40–49	50–59
Males	1200	2700	4200	3200
Females	1200	2700	4200	3200

Source: reference *73*.

Table 89

Annual prevalence of severe back pain per 100 000 population in the United Kingdom, 1987–1988

	Age groups (years)			
	20–29	30–39	40–49	50–59
Males	3100	4800	3000	4700
Females	3100	4800	3000	4700

Source: reference *73*.

Eastern Mediterranean Region — B

Table 90

Annual prevalence of severe back pain per 100 000 population in Oman, 1987

	Age groups (years)					
	16–25	26–35	36–45	46–55	56–65	≥65
Males	13 500	17 000	35 000	40 500	50 000	27 500
Females	26 000	47 000	54 000	52 500	50 000	41 000

Source: reference *77*.

Lifetime prevalence of experiencing back pain

Region of the Americas — A

Table 91

Lifetime prevalence of back pain per 100 000 population in the USA, 1992

	Age group (years)
	12–15
Males	27 970
Females	32 830

Source: reference *78*.

South-East Asia Region — B

Table 92

Lifetime prevalence of back pain per 100 000 population in Thailand, 1997

	Age group (years)
	≥15
Males	27 700
Females	27 000

Source: reference *79*.

South-East Asia Region — D

Table 93

Lifetime prevalence of back pain[a] per 100 000 population in India, 1988

	Age group (years)
	15–44
Males	19 000
Females	—

[a] Low back pain of more than 10 separate episodes.
Source: reference *70*.

European Region — A

Table 94

Lifetime prevalence of back pain per 100 000 population in Belgium, 1991

	Age groups (years)				
	15–19	20–34	35–49	50–64	≥65
Males	45 120	53 760	57 600	60 480	30 720
Females	48 880	58 240	62 400	65 520	66 560

Source: reference *80*.

Table 95

Lifetime prevalence of back pain[a] per 100 000 population in Denmark, 1998

	Age group (years)
	13–16
Males	49 800
Females	67 400

[a] Low back pain.
Source: reference *51*.

Table 96

Lifetime prevalence of back pain per 100 000 population in Sweden, 1994

	Age groups (years)		
	77–79	80–84	≥85
Males	9800	13 300	13 600
Females	22 100	16 900	14 800

Source: reference *72*.

Eastern Mediterranean Region — D

Table 97
Lifetime prevalence of back pain per 100 000 population in Pakistan, 1997

	Age band (years)
	≥15
Males	13 000
Females	26 000

Source: reference *81*.

Western Pacific Region — A

Table 98
Lifetime prevalence of back pain[a] per 100 000 population in Japan, 1977

	Age groups (years)				
	19	20–24	25–29	30–34	≥35
Males	61 800	69 700	62 006	52 300	70 000
Females	54 000	62 800	55 900	66 700	66 600

[a] Low back pain in supermarket workers.
Source: reference *82*.

Table 99
Lifetime prevalence of back pain[a] per 100 000 population in Japan, 1992

	Age groups (years)				
	<20	20–29	30–39	40–49	50–59
Males	49 300	56 700	64 300	69 800	63 500
Females	42 100	45 700	51 400	50 200	39 700

[a] Low back pain.
Source: reference *55*.

Table 100
Lifetime prevalence of back pain per 100 000 population in New Zealand, 1992

	Age groups (years)		
	<35	35–45	>45
Males	60 700	57 500	57 000
Females	64 700	61 200	60 900

Source: reference *57*.

Western Pacific Region — B

Table 101

Lifetime prevalence of back pain[a] per 100000 population in Beijing, China, 1992

	Age groups (years)					
	15–19	20–29	30–39	40–49	50–59	≥60
Males	14000	25000	22500	28000	38000	31000
Females	15000	28000	31500	52000	50000	51500

[a] Only low back pain reported above; neck and thoracic pain was noted in 3.3% of males and 7.0% of females in the population studied.

Source: reference *83*.

Table 102

Lifetime prevalence of back pain[a] per 100000 population in Hong Kong SAR, China, 1994

	Age groups (years)						
	<20	20–29	30–39	40–49	50–59	60–69	≥70
Males	8000	33000	18000	7000	14000	20000	4000
Females	10000	39000	33000	13000	24000	21000	12000

[a] Low back pain (16.7% of all males and females aged 20–59 reported pain lasting four or more weeks).

Source: reference *36*.

Lifetime prevalence of back pain that is severe or frequent or lasts more than seven days

Region of the Americas — A

Table 103

Lifetime prevalence of severe back pain[a] per 100000 population in the USA, 1988–1994

	Age groups (years)		
	18–44	45–64	≥65
Males	19900	30100	28200
Females	19900	30100	28800

[a] Back pain on most days for one month or more.

Source: reference *84*.

Table 104

Lifetime prevalence of severe back pain per 100000 population in the USA, 1992

	Age band (years)
	12–15
Males	6700
Females	8000

Source: reference *78*.

European Region — A

Table 105
Lifetime prevalence of severe back pain[a] per 100 000 population in the United Kingdom, 1992

	Age groups (years)			
	20–29	30–39	40–49	50–59
Males	8200	12 600	20 800	23 100
Females	7700	13 100	16 400	15 800

[a] Low back pain associated with a disability score of 9 or more.
Source: reference *85*.

European Region — B

The Scientific Group did not identify a data set from European Region — B and therefore suggested using the following data set from Greece.

Table 106
Lifetime prevalence of severe back pain[a] per 100 000 population in Greece

	Age groups (years)					
	19–28	29–38	39–48	49–58	59–68	>68
Males	1557	4902	11 494	9335	7143	4991
Females	1593	5781	12 182	10 881	10 534	7778

[a] Self-reported chronic back pain.
Source: reference *86*.

Eastern Mediterranean Region — B

The Scientific Group did not identify a data set from Eastern Mediterranean Region — B and therefore suggested using the following data set from Greece.

Table 107
Lifetime prevalence of severe back pain[a] per 100 000 population in Greece

	Age groups (years)					
	19–28	29–38	39–48	49–58	59–68	>68
Males	1557	4902	11 494	9335	7143	4991
Females	1593	5781	12 182	10 881	10 534	7778

[a] Self-reported chronic back pain.
Source: reference *86*.

Western Pacific Region — A

Table 108

Lifetime prevalence of severe back pain[a] per 100 000 population in Japan, 1977

	Age groups (years)				
	19	20–24	25–29	30–34	≥35
Males	17 100	18 200	19 300	19 700	35 000
Females	9 600	19 600	20 000	—	33 300

[a] Low back pain in supermarket workers, its severity indicating a need for medical examination.
Source: reference *82*.

Western Pacific Region — B

Table 109

Lifetime prevalence of severe back pain[a] per 100 000 population in Shantou, China, 1992

	Age groups (years)					
	15–19	20–29	30–39	40–49	50–59	≥60
Males	2000	2500	5000	4500	5000	5500
Females	3000	3500	5500	5500	8000	6000

[a] Only low back pain reported above; neck and thoracic pain were noted in 0.7% of males and 0.5% of females of the population studied.
Source: reference *83*.

Limb trauma

African Region — D

Table 110

Prevalence of limb trauma per 100 000 population in Ghana, 1999

	Age groups (years)				
	0–4	5–14	15–44	45–59	≥60
Males	540	1320	2480	1960	2830
Females	560	880	1580	3620	3710

Source: reference *87*.

Region of the Americas — A

Table 111

Prevalence of limb trauma[a] per 100 000 population in the USA, 1996

	Age groups (years)									
	0–4	5–14	15–24	25–34	35–44	45–54	55–64	65–74	75–84	≥85
Males	55	110	127	88	49	53	68	12	36	0
Females	33	49	82	84	43	31	63	51	166	41

[a] Self-reported trauma, all limbs.
Source: reference *60*.

Table 112
Prevalence of limb trauma[a] per 100 000 population in the USA, 1996

	Age groups (years)									
	0–4	5–14	15–24	25–34	35–44	45–54	55–64	65–74	75–84	≥85
Males	101	161	301	279	255	238	259	392	1002	2956
Females	71	80	110	110	135	185	332	783	2264	5479

[a] Cases based on hospital discharges, all limbs.
Source: reference *88*.

Table 113
Prevalence of lower limb trauma[a] per 100 000 population in the USA, 1996

	Age groups (years)									
	0–4	5–14	15–24	25–34	35–44	45–54	55–64	65–74	75–84	≥85
Males	20	54	27	24	21	30	39	0	36	0
Females	0	15	41	52	11	15	16	28	35	0

[a] Self-reported trauma, lower limbs.
Source: Reference *60*.

Table 114
Prevalence of lower limb trauma[a] per 100 000 population in the USA, 1996

	Age groups (years)									
	0–4	5–14	15–24	25–34	35–44	45–54	55–64	65–74	75–84	≥85
Males	61	84	191	173	167	164	191	321	907	2762
Females	34	39	79	81	102	145	263	649	2000	5016

[a] Cases based on hospital discharges.
Source: reference *88*.

Table 115
Prevalence of upper limb trauma per 100 000 population in the USA, 1996

	Age groups (years)									
	0–4	5–14	15–24	25–34	35–44	45–54	55–64	65–74	75–84	≥85
Males	35	57	100	64	28	24	26	12	0	0
Females	33	34	41	32	31	16	47	23	131	47

[a] Self-reported trauma, upper limbs.
Source: reference *60*.

Table 116
Prevalence of upper limb trauma[a] per 100 000 population in the USA, 1996

	Age groups (years)									
	0–4	5–14	15–24	25–34	35–44	45–54	55–64	65–74	75–84	≥85
Males	40	77	110	106	87	75	67	71	95	194
Females	38	41	31	30	33	42	69	135	264	463

[a] Cases based on hospital discharges.
Source: reference *88*.

World Region

Table 117

Rates of extremity injuries per 100 000 population resulting from falls

	Established market economies	Former socialist economies of Europe	India	China	Other countries in Asia and Islands	Sub-Saharan Africa	Latin America and the Caribbean	Middle Eastern crescent
Males (years)								
0–4	432.49	1153.51	3155.53	2131.34	4886.71	1012.60	1227.93	1933.70
5–14	381.42	1444.56	8611.98	1028.82	3009.24	2556.84	2269.80	2421.90
15–44	269.64	760.41	413.91	365.40	813.33	561.96	476.91	316.26
45–59	384.88	817.36	613.36	367.88	692.92	425.68	465.12	251.60
60 and over	406.56	353.28	242.88	346.08	159.36	216.96	353.28	77.76
All males	390.96	943.20	2658.24	726.48	1939.68	1195.92	1020.96	121.77
Females (years)								
0–4	239.72	710.32	3016.00	2844.40	3295.76	977.60	699.92	1449.24
5–14	173.04	564.48	4288.20	973.56	1577.52	1705.20	1190.28	1145.76
15–44	166.32	378.84	572.04	269.64	557.76	381.36	267.96	201.60
45–49	626.56	1007.60	1695.76	1996.72	1176.56	626.56	619.52	384.56
60 and over	1622.72	1117.60	546.48	1628.00	265.76	858.00	990.88	175.12
All females	559.41	722.10	2220.24	1197.12	1476.39	1021.38	694.26	824.76
All	487.08	868.38	2576.44	973.34	1802.36	1160.30	907.74	1034.84

Source: reference *89*.

Table 118
Rates of extremity injuries per 100 000 population resulting from road traffic accidents

	Established market economies	Former socialist economies of Europe	India	China	Other countries in Asia and Islands	Sub-Saharan Africa	Latin America and the Caribbean	Middle Eastern crescent
Males (years)								
0–4	19.50	22.00	67.50	19.25	72.25	37.75	34.75	16.50
5–14	145.92	198.24	280.32	112.32	236.64	471.36	437.28	193.44
15–44	212.94	312.06	132.30	97.86	141.12	189.00	238.14	140.70
45–59	138.03	294.55	166.84	125.99	142.33	184.04	275.63	125.13
60 and over	95.20	108.64	83.44	79.24	74.20	94.08	143.08	49.28
All males	161.13	237.39	154.98	93.89	149.24	219.35	244.36	121.77
Females (years)								
0–4	17.69	15.95	23.78	17.11	79.46	30.45	31.32	17.11
5–14	59.20	68.80	143.68	75.20	87.68	152.64	150.40	63.36
15–44	107.63	59.22	37.13	33.37	39.48	54.05	80.37	25.85
45–49	53.24	72.16	97.68	66.88	54.56	50.60	78.76	33.44
60 and over	67.20	69.72	88.20	49.98	60.06	32.34	74.34	33.18
All females	79.64	65.12	84.04	48.84	70.40	91.96	102.52	41.80
All	119.70	148.68	120.96	72.24	110.46	155.82	173.88	83.16

Source: reference *89*.

References

1. **Arnett FC et al.** The American Rheumatism Association 1987 revised criteria for the classification of rheumatoid arthritis. *Arthritis and rheumatism*, 1988, **30**:315–324.
2. **Ropes MW et al.** Revision of diagnostic criteria for rheumatoid arthritis. *Bulletin on the rheumatic diseases*, 1958, **9**:175–176.
3. **Muller AS, Valkenburg HA, Greenwood BM.** Rheumatoid arthritis in three West African populations. *East African medical journal*, 1972, **49**:75–83.
4. **Moolenburgh JD, Valkenburg HA, Fourie PB.** A population study on rheumatoid arthritis in Lesotho, Southern Africa. *Annals of the rheumatic diseases*, 1986, **45**:691–695.
5. **Solomon L, Robin G, Valkenburg HA.** Rheumatoid arthritis in an urban South African Negro population. *Annals of the rheumatic diseases*, 1975, **34**:128–135.
6. **Beighton P, Solomon L, Valkenburg HA.** Rheumatoid arthritis in a rural South African population. *Annals of the rheumatic diseases*, 1975, **34**:136–141.
7. **Gabriel SE, Crowson CS, O'Fallon WM.** Juvenile rheumatoid arthritis in Rochester, Minnesota. 1955–1985. *Arthritis and rheumatism*, 1999, **42**:415–420.
8. **Peterson LS et al.** Juvenile rheumatoid arthritis in Rochester, Minnesota 1960–1993. Is the epidemiology changing? *Arthritis and rheumatism*, 1996, **39**:1385–1390.
9. **Lawrence JS et al.** Rheumatoid arthritis in a subtropical population. *Annals of the rheumatic diseases*, 1966, **25**:59–66.
10. **Darmawan J et al.** The epidemiology of rheumatoid arthritis in Indonesia. *British journal of rheumatology*, 1993, **32**:537–540.
11. **Kvien TK et al.** The prevalence and severity of rheumatoid arthritis in Oslo. *Scandinavian journal of rheumatology*, 1997, **26**:412–418.
12. **Gare BA, Fasth A.** Epidemiology of juvenile chronic arthritis in southwestern Sweden. *Pediatrics*, 1992, **90**:950–958.
13. **Tzonchev VT, Pilossoff T, Kanev K.** Prevalence of osteoarthritis in Bulgaria. In: Bennett PH, Wood PHN, eds. *Population studies of the rheumatic diseases. Proceedings of the third international symposium, New York 1966.* Amsterdam, Excerpta Medica, 1968:413–415.
14. **Khuffash FA, Majeed HA.** Juvenile rheumatoid arthritis among Arab children. *Scandinavian journal of rheumatology*, 1988, **17**:393–395.
15. **Al-Rawi ZS et al.** Rheumatoid arthritis in population samples in Iraq. *Annals of the rheumatic diseases*, 1978, **37**:73–75.
16. **Lau E et al.** Low prevalence of rheumatoid arthritis in the urbanized Chinese of Hong Kong. *Journal of rheumatology*, 1993, **20**:1133–1137.
17. **Beasley RP, Bennett PH, Lin CC.** Low prevalence of rheumatoid arthritis in Chinese: prevalence survey in a rural community. *Journal of rheumatology*, 1983, **10**(suppl. 10):11–15.

18. **Kellgren JH, Lawrence JS.** Osteoarthritis and disc degeneration in an urban population. *Annals of the rheumatic diseases*, 1958, **17**:388–397.

19. **Solomon L.** Osteoarthrosis in a rural South African Negro population. *Annals of the rheumatic diseases*, 1976, **35**:274.

20. **United States Department of Health, Education and Welfare.** *NHANES I: basic data on arthritis: knee, hip and sacro-iliac joints. Adults ages 25–74 years. United States 1971–1975.* Hyattsville, MD, USA, National Center for Health Statistics, 1979 (DHEW Publication No 79–1661, Vital and Health Statistics, Series 11, No. 213(8/79) (available at: *http://www.cdc.gov/nchs/data/series/sr_11/sr11_213.pdf*).

21. **Bremner JM, Lawrence JS, Miall WE.** Degenerative joint disease in a Jamaican rural population. *Annals of the rheumatic diseases*, 1968, **27**:326–32. Cited in Lawrence JS, Sebo M. The geography of osteoarthrosis. In: Nuki G, ed. *The aetiopathogenesis of osteoarthrosis.* Tunbridge Wells, Pitman Medical, 1980:155–182.

22. **Danielsson L, Lindberge H.** Prevalence of coxarthrosis in an urban population during four decades. *Clinical orthopaedics and related research*, 1997, **342**:106–110.

23. **Tzonchev VT, Pilossoff T, Kanev K.** Prevalence of osteoarthritis in Bulgaria. In: Bennett PH, Wood PHN, eds. *Population studies of the rheumatic diseases. Proceedings of the third international symposium, New York 1966.* Amsterdam, Excerpta Medica, 1968:413–415.

24. **Pogrund H et al.** Osteoarthritis of the hip joint and osteoporosis: a radiological study in a random population sample in Jerusalem. *Clinical orthopaedics and related research*, 1982, **164**:130–135.

25. **Ota H.** Prevalence of osteoarthrosis of the hip and other joints in Japanese population. *Journal of the Japanese Orthopaedic Association*, 1979, **53**:165–180.

26. **Hoaglund FT, Yau,AC, Wong WL.** Osteoarthritis of the hip and other joints in Southern Chinese in Hong Kong. *Journal of bone and joint surgery*, 1973, **55A**:545–557.

27. **Solomon L, Beighton P, Lawrence JS.** Rheumatic disorders in the South African Negro. II. Osteoarthrosis. *South African medical journal*, 1975, **49**:1737–1740.

28. **Davis MA et al.** Sex differences in osteoarthritis of the knee. *American journal of epidemiology*, 1988, **127**:1019–1030.

29. **Felson DT.** Epidemiology of hip and knee osteoarthritis. *Epidemiology reviews*, 1988, **10**:1–28.

30. **Valkenburg HA.** Clinical versus radiological osteoarthrosis in the general population. In: Peyron JG, ed. *Epidemiology of osteoarthritis.* Paris, Geigy, 1980:53–58.

31. **Altman R et al.** Development of criteria for the classification and reporting of osteoarthritis: classification of osteoarthritis of the knee. *Arthritis and rheumatism*, 1986, **29**:1039–1049.

32. **Carmona L, Laffon A for the EPISER Study Group.** The prevalence of 6 rheumatic diseases in the Spanish population. *Annals of the rheumatic diseases*, 2000, **59**(suppl. 1):67.

33. **Gibson T et al.** Knee pain amongst the poor and affluent in Pakistan. *British journal of rheumatology*, 1996, **35**:146–149.

34. **Tamaki M, Koga Y.** Osteoarthritis of the knee joint: a field study. *Journal of the Japanese Orthopaedic Association*, 1994, 68:737–750.

35. **Adebajo AO, Cooper C, Evans JG.** Fractures of the hip and distal forearm in West Africa and the United Kingdom. *Age and ageing*, 1991, **20**:435–438.

36. **Solomon L.** Osteoporosis and fracture of the femoral neck in the South African Bantu. *Journal of bone and joint surgery*, 1968, **50B**:2–13.

37. **Melton LJ III, Crowson CS, O'Fallon WM.** Fracture incidence in Olmsted County, Minnesota: comparison of urban with rural rates and changes in urban rates over time. *Osteoporosis international*, 1999, **9**:29–37.

38. **Schwartz AV et al.** International variation in the incidence of hip fractures: cross-national project on osteoporosis for the World Health Organization Program for Research on Aging. *Osteoporosis international*, 1999, 9:242–253.

39. **Bacon WE et al.** International comparison of hip fractures in 1988–89. *Osteoporosis international*, 1996, 6:69–75.

40. **Lau E et al.** The incidence of hip fractures in five Asian countries — the Asian Osteoporosis Study (AOS). *Osteoporosis international*, 2001, **12**:239–243.

41. **Rowe SM, Yoon TR, Ryang DH.** An epidemiological study of hip fracture in Honam, Korea. *International orthopaedics*, 1993, **17**:139–143.

42. **European Communities.** *Report on osteoporosis in the European Community: action for prevention.* Luxembourg, Office for Official Publications of the European Communities, 1998.

43. **Elffors I et al.** The variable incidence of hip fracture in southern Europe: the MEDOS study. *Osteoporosis international*, 1994, **4**:253–263.

44. **Schwartz AV et al.** International variation in the incidence of hip fractures: cross-national project on osteoporosis for the World Health Organization Program for Research on Ageing. *Osteoporosis international*, 1999, **9**:242–253.

45. **Memon A et al.** Incidence of hip fracture in Kuwait. *International journal of epidemiology*, 1998, **27**:860–865.

46. **Sanders KM et al.** Age- and gender-specific rate of fractures in Australia: a population-based study. *Osteoporosis international*, 1999, **10**:240–247.

47. **Cobb JR.** Outline for the study of scoliosis. In: Edwards JW, ed. *Instructional course lectures.* Ann Arbor, MI, American Academy of Orthopaedic Surgeons, 1948, **5**:261–275

48. **Weinstein SL.** Natural history. *Spine*, 1999, **24**:2592–2600.

49. **Mulimba JO.** The problems of low back pain in Africa. *East African medical journal*, 1990, **67**:250–253.

50. **Darmawan J et al.** The prevalence of soft tissue rheumatism in Indonesia — a WHO–ILAR COPCORD Study. *Rheumatology international*, 1995, **15**:121–124.

51. **Harreby M et al.** Risk factors for low back pain in a cohort of 1389 Danish school children: an epidemiological study. *European spine journal*, 1999, 8:444–450.

52. **Reigo T, Timpka T, Tropp H.** The epidemiology of back pain in vocational age groups. *Scandinavian journal of primary health care*, 1999, **17**:17–21.

53. *The prevalence of back pain in Great Britain in 1998.* London, Government Statistical Service, 1999 (Crown Bulletin, No. 18).

54. **Armenian HK, Halabi SS, Khlat M.** Epidemiology of primary health problems in Beirut. *Journal of epidemiology and community health*, 1989, **43**: 315–318.

55. **Matsui H et al.** Risk indicators of low back pain among workers in Japan. *Spine*, 1997, **22**:1242–1248.

56. **Laslett M et al.** The frequency and incidence of low back pain/sciatica in an urban population. *New Zealand medical journal*, 1991, **104**:424–426.

57. **Coggan C et al.** Prevalence of back pain among nurses. *New Zealand medical journal*, 1994, **107**:306–308.

58. **Manahan L et al.** Rheumatic pain in a Philippine village. A WHO–ILAR COPCORD study. *Rheumatology international*, 1985, **5**:149–153.

59. **Worku Z.** Prevalence of low back pain in Lesotho mothers. *Journal of manipulative and physiological therapeutics*, 2000, **23**:147–154.

60. **Adams PF, Hendershot, GE, Maranao MA.** *Current estimates, from the National Health Interview Survey, 1996.* Hyattsville, MD, National Center for Health Statistics, 1999 (Vital and Health Statistics Series 10, No. 200. DHHS Publication No (PHS) 99–1528) (available at: *http://www.cdc.gov/nchs/data/series/sr_10/sr10_200.pdf*).

61. **Leboeuf-Yde C, Kyvik KO.** At what age does low back pain become a common problem? *Spine*, 1998, **23**:228–234.

62. **Svensson HO, Andersson GB.** Low back pain in forty to forty-seven year old men. I. Frequency of occurrence and impact on medical services. *Scandinavian journal of rehabilitation medicine*, 1982, **14**:47–53.

63. **Chahade WH.** *Multicentric studies of the prevalence of adult rheumatoid arthritis and low back pain in Brazilian adult population samples.* São Paulo, Hospital do Servidor Publico Estadual de São Paulo, 1999.

64. **Svensson HO et al.** A retrospective study of low-back pain in 38- to 64-year-old women. *Spine*, 1988, **13**:548–552.

65. **Australian Bureau of Statistics.** *1995 National Health Survey: Summary of Results.* Canberra, Australian Government Printing Service, 1995 (ABS Catalogue No. 4364.0).

66. **Schierhout GH, Meyers JE, Bridger RS.** Work related musculoskeletal disorders and ergonomic stressors In the South African workforce. *Occupational and environmental medicine*, 1995, **52**:46–50.

67. **Bressler HB et al.** The prevalence of low back pain in the elderly. A systematic review of the literature. *Spine*, 1999, **24**:1813–1819.

68. **Sternbach RA.** Survey of pain in the United States: the Nuprin Pain Report. *Clinical journal of pain*, 1986, **2**:49–53.

69. **Edmond SL, Felson DT.** Prevalence of back symptoms in elders. *Journal of rheumatology*, 2000, **7**:220–225.

70. **Ory FG, Rahman FU, Katagade V et al.** Respiratory disorders, skin complaints and low-back trouble among tannery workers in Kanpur, India. *American Industrial Hygiene Association journal*, 1997, **58**:740–746.

71. **Anderson RT.** An orthopedic ethnography in rural Nepal. *Medical anthropology*, 1984, **8**:46–59.

72. **Brattberg G, Parker MG, Thorslund M.** The prevalence of pain among the oldest old in Sweden. *Pain*, 1996, **67**:29–34.

73. **Palmer KT et al.** Back pain in Britain: comparison of two prevalence surveys at an interval of 10 years. *British medical journal*, 2000, **320**:1577–1579.

74. **Wigley RD et al.** Rheumatic complaints in Tokelau. *Rheumatology international*, 1987, **7**:61–65.

75. **Reisbord LS, Greenland S.** Factors associated with self-reported back pain prevalence: a population-based study. *Journal of chronic disease*, 1985, **38**:691–702.

76. **Santos-Eggimann B et al.** One-year prevalence of low back pain in two Swiss regions. *Spine*, 2000, **25**:2473–2479.

77. **Pountain G.** Musculoskeletal pain in Omanis, and the relationship to joint mobility and body mass index. *British journal of rheumatology*, 1992, **31**:81–85.

78. **Olsen TL et al.** The epidemiology of low back pain in an adolescent population. *American journal of public health*, 1992, **82**:606–608.

79. **Chaiamnuay P et al.** Epidemiology of rheumatic disease in Thailand: a WHO–ILAR COPCORD Study. *Journal of rheumatology*, 1998, **25**:1382–1387.

80. **Skovron ML et al.** Sociocultural factors and low back pain. *Spine*, 1994, **19**:129–137.

81. **Farooqi A, Gibson T.** Prevalence of the major rheumatic disorders in the adult population of North Pakistan. *British journal of rheumatology*, 1998, **37**:491–495.

82. **Ohmichi A, Abuku S, Kataoka C.** Complaints of low back pain among the workers of supermarkets. *Sangyo igaku* [*Japanese journal of industrial health*], 1977, **19**:94–95.

83. **Wigley RD et al.** Rheumatic disease in China: ILAR–China study comparing the prevalence of rheumatic symptoms in northern and southern rural populations. *Journal of rheumatology*, 1994, **21**:1484–1490.

84. **Praemer A, Furner S, Rice DP.** *Musculoskeletal conditions in the United States*. Rosemont, IL, American Academy of Orthopaedic Surgeons, 1999.

85. **Walsh K, Cruddas M, Coggon D.** Low back pain in eight areas of Britain. *Journal of epidemiology and community health*, 1992, **46**:227–230.

735

86. **Georgountoz A et al.** Prevalence of low back pain in urban, suburban and rural population in Greece. *Annals of the rheumatic diseases*, 2000, **59**(suppl. 1):218.

87. **Mock CN et al.** Incidence and outcome of injury in Ghana: results of a community based survey. *Bulletin of the World Health Organization*, 1999, **77**:955–964.

88. **Agency for Healthcare Research and Quality.** *Nationwide inpatient sample.* Rockville, MD, 2000 (available at: http://www.ahrq.gov/data/hcup/hcupnis.htm).

89. **Murray CJL, Lopez AD.** *Global health statistics.* Geneva, World Health Organization, 1996 (Global Burden of Disease and Injury Series, Vol. II).